If I Am
Must Be

Horace Smith

chipmunkapublishing
the mental health publisher

Horace Smith

Published by
Chipmunkapublishing
PO Box 6872
Brentwood
Essex CM13 1ZT
United Kingdom

http://www.chipmunkapublishing.com

Chipmunkapublishing gratefully acknowledge the support of Arts Council England.

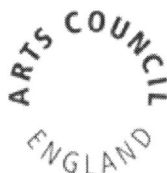

If I Am Then I Must Be

Chapter 1

Therefore, remember to understand this book of abstract thoughts, poetical forms of literature, idioms speeches, and parables you must first be a liberated intellectual theorist, and thinker. And you must look at them as a reflection of who you are, and not who I am. Look at them as you would, when you look into the mirror in the mornings to remember what you look like. If there is some verse or maybe a whole chapter that you do not understand, then stop reading and examine your conscience to see what you have hidden there in the dark that I have brought to the light. And so let me begin as I introduce myself to you, my full name is, 'Horace James Smith,' 'Horace,' meaning, 'Light of The Sun,' and my name's spiritual connotation is, 'Victorious Spirit.' Also 'Horace,' means, 'Keeper of Time,' so in a sense I am a, 'Time Lord,' like, 'Doctor Who,' the first black British with Indian and African blood in me as my consciousness was created over four continents that is Asia, Africa, the Caribbean that is Jamaica and the UK and over a six thousand period of years.

From one generation to the next from one mother to the next until I am that I am. And that is the sum of all the experiences from Eve the first woman ever created by Christ to me. I transcend time and space by my schizophrenia, which is my Tardis and that, is by perception I can look at an object in most cases in fantasy films and plot their course back through time and in some cases look at their future as you will see in this book. Like for instance, 'Charles Darwin's Tree of Life,' it began in the, 'Garden of Eden,' as the, 'Tree of Life and the Tree of The Knowledge of God and Evil,' we see it resurface in the most recent remake of the fantasy flick called, '300,' where the Spartan, hence if you were to take out of the, 'P and the R,' you will have the word 'Satan,' so in a sense the word, 'Spartan is a code name for those who are Satan's little helpers and do not even know it, but as I was saying, and the, 'P,' and 'R,' is an abbreviation for p. r. stunt. 'The Tree of the Knowledge of Good and Evil and The Tree of Life and Death,' is seen in clear view as in the dark from a far distance, away as all the King's men look on in horror as they see what Xerxes did by hanging the dead bodies of the poor innocent villagers on the tree. 'The Tree of the Knowledge of Good and Evil and Life and Death,' hence 'Charles Darwin's Tree of Life,' and 'The two trees found in the Garden of Eden,' 'the Tree of life and the Tree of the Knowledge of Good and Evil,' and the Tree that Christ was hanged on and died on it and the Tree the many Black African Americans were lynched on, where Conan the Barbarian that is Arnold Schwarzenegger was hanged on, a enormous tree and left to die by James Earl Jones.

In addition, here it is use to make commerce for the Beast of the Ancient Egyptian Empire's commerce in slave labor. And as you read about this journey on the road called going to a destination called nowhere, that I call life and life to me is like a small little child who has just learnt to walk and thus begins his journey in his newly acquired skills that is walking of course, as he begins his walking journey that leads to a dead end street, he walks on and on and on and on and so he continues to walk, but yet he is getting nowhere, as he reaches his teenage years, he is still walking on that same path leading to a dead end street, it is called the journey of getting old and never really changing, never really being aware of what he is becoming and what he has already become and really never living in the freedom that is all around him, because he is told he must continue to walk to get to his destination, which cannot be found because it does not exist and so he is told, if he is late for work he will be deducted money from his pay check for the work not done, and if he continues to be late getting to his place of employment he will be terminated, he is told he must continue walking if he wants to get home to watch a little television, eat his evening meal, then retire to his bed, to begin the same journey again, the next day and that is to walk in the same foot steps of those who have taken this journey before but never returned, and when he becomes an adult, and has gone through a mid life crises, he continues to walk, and so as he begins to get old and frail, he is still walking on the road to nowhere, and then one day he is seen no more, walking this lonely road of going nowhere, for you see to move from one point in the road to your destination in time to another you must perceive differently and so your perception and awareness must change and grow.

And then you will see that it is not the walking the same path in the journey of life all our lives that matters but however, it is our perception of our life's journey on that walking journey to nowhere that changes us as we perceive perception, and as we think we create ourselves, which is a mirrored image of what we think we are, the personified image of perception, 'If I am then I must be,' and so as we are on that walking journey going to a destination called nowhere, and as we learn to be content and enjoy it a little more, as we walk to our graves, where all roads leads and where all journeys must end, that is in the Holy city of the Roman Empire, for all walks on the path of life must end and cease to exist in the land of perception, as the night quickly approaches and so we begin to exist in the abyss of darkness where time is still, where there is no light to see and is ever quiet, that is the road, it is called hell on earth, the region of the damned coming out of the earth, to haunt me, it is the road that I was born on, and have been on for the last 45 years of my life, which will help you to see why the nurse at Saint Thomas Hospital in Lambeth on the 19th October 1964, by the river Thames institutionally named me so, and William Shakespeare was born 1564.

So let me give you a brief summary of my former life and its history. At the age of ten I was sodomized in a horrendous act of sodomy, by two power hungry black Jamaican Catholic priests, who made a covenant with the devil the God of my ancestors Olorun the God of the Yoruba people of West Africa, to gain much mind controlling power, the kind you see those, practiced by witchdoctors on the dark ancient continent of Africa, the ancient oasis in the desert sands of distance lands, a place of diversity, a place of dark magic and intrigue, where the People come in all shapes and sizes, with some unseen differences in their abilities and appearances. In addition, so throughout the history of this ancient Dark Continent come many different faces of Man now found throughout the world. Even though the faces takes on different shapes and sizes, different shades of black, the genetic structure, the DNA, remains the same indifferent to what most people are taught to believe.

Therefore, about 99% of the DNA in all humanity is similar in identity, which is not an accident. For the most part, the protein that carries out the biochemical function of a human body was made the same from one person to the next. The remaining one percent, however, accounts for people's diversity. It can also be used as a tool to determine how genetically related people are. This oneness is of all races is an interest to the curiously nosey minded, ever since DNA was discovered and how it now functions in certain patterns. These nosey parkers thought that perhaps the study of DNA could provide the essential clues in the long-standing quest for an understanding of the evolution of Homo sapiens. A stumbling block in walking on the road called going nowhere for when one who takes this mundane journey, becomes bored with the journey, his instincts for being nosey compels him to continue when, the silent voice of conscience and intuition tells him not to continue, but his thirst to be an intellectual of sorts, forces him that is the expression of the mind, controlling all bodily functions, the voice of reason, to continue down this dark path on the road called going nowhere, for he searches for the has been of the basic process of meiosis, a process commonly known to biologist as the process of cell division in organisms that reproduce sexually as cells divides during that which is called the nucleus divides into nuclei, with each one continuing in half the usual number of chromosomes the recombination of the genetic factors from both the male and female of the species called by himself Homo sapiens.

However, there is one form of DNA that is inherited from only the female; thus going back as far as being traced back in time, to the one and only, 'the ancestor of us all,' her name is called Eve, the mother of the living, who first began this journey on the road called going nowhere, when she consumed with lust the Apple of conscience. Hence, the nosey parkers have coined up the "Eve Theory," that all life originated from Africa, that mysteriously dark ancient continent. My grandmother's place of birth, but in her wisdom she fled that ancient dark continent of mysticism, which is that ancient question that morality that is the new and improve moral conscience of the Homo sapiens, the spiritual children of thought that allowed Hitlerism to built on one of the side roads, adjacent to the main road called going nowhere, the concept of the Superman syndrome.

A Super race of Superhuman morality, formerly known as the Third Reich, or more to the point the Aryan nation or more bluntly, the Nazi ideology, belonging to or having the characteristics of the fictitious Aryan race, a phonetically sounded syllable of the mid 19th century formed from Sanskrit arya, of nobility of good family, originally a national name denoting the worshippers of the gods of the Brahmans from the Indo European. A word denoting Lord Ruler, as we now see in the west, the hero complex. "The perfect man who is a good person, a moral character, an exceptional man, a man possessing exceptional strength, abilities and powers, Nietzsche' ideal man, according to the philosophy of Nietzsche, an ideal man who through creativity and integrity is able to transcend good and evil and is the goal of human evolution, but without mercy, compassion and true justice," by not going down the wrong path in the journey of human understanding the school of human intellect, knowledge without wisdom to use it wisely.

As Henry the Satanist priest in the disguise of the Roman Catholic black Jamaican Church tried to suffocate me as he penetrated me, and tried turn me into Satan's whore bride, as in the movie called, 'Bride of Dracula,' in what he called his satanic ritual service, which when later I talked to my Doctors about they could not answer the question, maybe it was too horrible to think that men could do such horrible things to a child, because that child is weak and defenseless, as they like spiritual sexual vampires, feed on the virtue of an innocent child, as I am only ten, as they turned me into a walking undead, not seen by anyone, not known by anyone but what they think is their victory by stealing my virtue, as they gain more power by my ruminating on the fact that they have penetrated me, a ten year old child and stolen my innocence.

They know that I will never have any true friends, that I will never marry, that I will never be able to hold down a good job, and that all my thinking life will be about what they did to me, and why they did what they did to me, in the hope that I would go out and do what they did, but however, I was one step ahead of them, because I was an intelligent child, and knew, even at that age that what had happened was very serious, and that I needed to isolate myself so that I could contain the infection, and so while in America I would not socialize with anyone who was on the road going to nowhere, as I knew that I would have ended up like those on the chat shows who feel that they have been conned, as they are lied to by our leaders who have made a contract with the road going to nowhere, to bring them many souls with their false information, that are full of lies and half truths. I remained isolated until I found out why I was sodomized in a satanic ritual ceremony, and that was for the Satanist to make a host to put all the knowledge of William Shakespeare, and Hitler into me. As I was hallucinating in my room in Boston hearing voices, screaming at me, that in a past life I was Hitler, but when I got back to London, and after many years of therapy, and I was well enough, and not so much in shock of the whole event, that took place in Boston I began to look into the names of Hitler and William Shakespeare, and the connection to my name is the abbreviation, 'HRE,' as in the, 'Holy Roman Empire.' I also found out that in Psalm 46 in the King James Bible, you find the sign post of Shakespeare's name.

In verse, three you find the word, 'Shake,' and in verse nine you will find the word, 'Spear,' when added together you get Shakespeare. Now if you were to take the chapter of this Psalm, which is 46, and invert it you get the year that I was born that is 64 and if you were to go further and add the 4 and 6, you will get the numeral 10, which is the month that I was born, then add the numeral 10, to the numeral 9, you will get the numeral 19, the day and century that I was born. Kind of like an Omen - Daemon type of scenario in my life. However, if you were to subtract the numeral 3 from the numeral 19 you will get the numeral 16 hence the 16th Century where I think Shakespeare was born, (1564.) But the truth is both Henry and Harry I forgave a long time ago, for what they did and that was to destroy my life, but yet Henry is dead and Harry, I have no idea where he is but they went on to live their lives, while I suffered the shame and disgrace, and most importantly the isolation that was meant for them in life.

In fact, I learnt a long time ago that life is not just or fair. Life is what you make of it, and if you do not have the right answers you will live the wrong life, as you see many on those daytime chat shows do, as you listen to the horror stories of going down the dead end street, that leads to nowhere, and as they sit and air their pains, frustrations, there is no one to tell them that they had gone down a road that leads to nowhere, and what they are revealing is the sum of all they have experienced from traveling the journey to nowhere, the endless regret, the delusional state of living for nothing but a nightmare for all their lives, and now that they think that their lives

If I Am Then I Must Be

are almost over, they are bitter and they strike out at anyone who they see on that road going to nowhere, that we all must travel at one time or another until most of us find a purpose to live for other than to control others, because we think that we are important, when in truth our conscience is speaking to us, telling us that we are on a road to nowhere, and so we fight it, the voices of our heart, that is intuition for our foolish pride, and we continuing down the road to nowhere, trying to control others, and I know, because I have done it myself. However, some like me eventually see the light, in the dark, so that I can recognize the dark in the light, when I come off that road that leads to nowhere, and hopefully in the process, open the eyes of many who can see me on the road going to nowhere.

When they see that, I am no longer traveling the same road to nowhere, and then they wonder where I have gone, and so begin to pursue me. The true condition of humanity without a conscience but instead the only a God who speaks for this, the God of our ancestors, which led us into slavery, and sexual immorality, and cannibalism, and so much more horrid ways of the expression of mind, hence now called the intellectual stimulus, that is has now evolved into a thought made real it is called mental illness, in my case schizophrenia, thus reminding me, by showing me, that I have chosen the wrong path by reminding me of my injuries in the walking the broad path leading nowhere, instead of walking the straight and narrow path, that leads somewhere, and that is the inner conflict manifested on the outside from the imagination to my own deluded perception, that everyone is my enemy, which is one of the main symptoms of this creation of the id called the Frankenstein monster, that has come to life it is called schizophrenia, yes I did not know the depths of the darkness, that I was seeing, walking on the road called going nowhere, seeing the death and destruction, that my African ancestor Olorun, Olorun the God of the Yoruba people of West Africa, the myth, he was the wisest of the Gods, and was the supreme ruler of the sky, hence the forerunner of the intellectual Homo sapiens.

Yes, my grandmother wisely embarked on a spiritual experience, and went to Jamaica, where she married an Indian from India, and has now ceased to walk on that ancient path going to a place called nowhere, where all must go, for many centuries. It has existed and yet no one has discovered its intentions. And those who came close to understanding this ancient path that leads to nowhere, were executed by lane of curiosity, like John F. Kennedy, Martin Luther King Jr., Gandhi, Abraham Lincoln, and the most famous of them all Jesus Christ, who came back to life, from that destination on the road called going nowhere ends, and in so leaving behind that ancient road called going nowhere. Hence showing the way, that leads in the opposite direction from the road called going nowhere to the road called, 'and let this mind be in you, which was also in Jesus who, being in the form of God, thought it not robbery to be equal with God but made himself of no reputation and took upon him the form of a servant, and was made in the likeness of men: and being found in fashion as a man he humbled himself and became obedient unto death and even the death of the cross. Wherefore God also hath highly exalted him, and given him a name, which is above every name: that at the name of Jesus every knee should bow of things in heaven, and things in the earth and things under the earth; and that every tongue should confess that Jesus is Lord to the glory of God the Father.'

I call it hypnosis, that is used to make money and gain fame, at the expense of destroying a child's virtue and innocence, that is my innocence, as I am penetrated, and wounded before marriage, like a white angelic virgin, before her wedding day is violated, because she could not wait for her, 'Prince Charming,' my, 'Prince Charming,' would have been a good education, maybe even Oxford or Cambridge University, then onto a great career, as a professional, and then to fall in love with my childhood sweet heart, then marriage, then would have came the children, a nice home, and a nice car but non of this happened, it was all stolen from me or so would one think, but in truth because I did not give up in my hope of my life being restored I am about to enter my, 'Promised Land,' my 'Canaan,' a different, 'Canaan Land,' as we are brainwashed into believing in the school of thoughts, where fantasies are lived out, it is called, 'The School of a Fallen Life,' the place where we learn about our past to build the future, and in the academic sense of the word, four plus four will always equal eight, hence by learning about the past, we only create the past in our futures, the answer to a riddle a once wise man announced, as he went on this journey to nowhere, 'that history always repeats itself,' because as a Homo

If I Am Then I Must Be

sapiens thinks, so is a Homo sapiens, but if you meditate on it for a while, and listen to your intuition speaking to you through your conscience, saying, 'if we study the past will we not create the past in the present future?' And the betting office of life, on the road called going nowhere, always wins, because they understand, and know that the past will always repeat itself and so it is a safe bet, a guaranteed winner.

And so it was in my mother's church, in a satanic ritual, as I was their host, at the age of ten to breed all kinds of mind controlling drugs of power, like that which hypnotist uses to control people's minds and lives, I call it parapsychology, then they handed me over to a pedophile ring to be constantly abused, it is called the ring of self perceptions, and so I grew up believing in a lie, that I was abused by two black Jamaican Catholic priests, and that I was a wounded child, growing into a man, but in truth I abused myself, because I believed the lies, and fables about growing up with abuse like the ancient people believed in their idols, based on their superstitions, and so they became slaves to a dead way of life, the walking dead, as the apostle Paul once wrote about two thousand years ago, as he said, 'to beware lest any man spoil you through philosophy and vain deceit, after the tradition of men, after the rudiments of the world, and not after Christ For in Christ dwelleth all the fullness of the Godhead bodily. And ye are complete in him, which is the head of all principality and power: In whom also ye are circumcised with the circumcision made without hands, in putting off the body of the sins of the flesh by the circumcision of Christ the Christ: buried with him in baptism, wherein also ye are risen with him through the faith of the dead. And you, being dead in your sins and the uncircumcision of your flesh, hath he quickened together with him, having forgiven you all your trespasses; Blotting out the handwriting of ordinances and traditions that were past down from generation to generation that kept our future children living our great grandparent's failures as individuals and as a society in whole, which is still against us, which is still contrary to us, and took it out of the way, nailing it to his cross; and having spoiled principalities and powers, he made a shew of them openly, triumphing over them in it. Let no man therefore judge you in meat, or in drink, or in respect of holyday, or of the new moon, (when werewolves are seen and Count Dracula the Prince of Darkness comes out to play with his toy dolls of porcelain,) or of the Sabbath days: which is the shadow of things to come; but the body is of Christ Let no man beguile you of your reward in a voluntary humility and worshipping of angels, intruding into those things which he hath not seen vainly puffed up by his fleshly mind.'

And so not being able to smell the fresh morning winter breeze in the golden winter sun, and all its goodness, or watch the stars, as they blink in the starry eyed sea of passionate dark blue nights, it is it called the traditions of our forefathers, as we honor the death of those gone forever, that we seemed to can't let go of, and so out a sense of duty, and loyalty they follow an ancient practice of honoring the dead, that has no bearing or relevance to modern day life, and that is finding the truth, the way and the path that leads to life, and freedom from a mental slavery, that is if, 'I am then I must be,' and the hidden truth of this saying found at the end of the journey on the road called going nowhere, which is, and then to be no more, for all must die forgotten, like a man who forgets what he looks like after leaving his mirror behind, that is the mirror of his perception of his life, that is his ego or more rather his little id becoming a big id like, a big head who knows it all but yet has accomplished nothing in life, because you can't take it with you, as the Pharaohs thought they could, so they were buried with their slaves, and gold to serve them in the after life, and so what a waste of life to satisfy the little id now, a big id thus controlling a nation in one's folly, and that is that fallen man is God, as the honorable gentlemen would denote in his proclamation of the failed experiment called the Labour party, the Conservatives, the Liberal democrats sitting down in a room of debates, and endless self admiration of each others' ego, thus stroking the little id, being perplexed in the debate, "why isn't our government working, and so lets change it," and so another government comes in with the same old debates and that is, "why isn't it working, and lets change it," and tries for another eight years to make an ideal that does not exist, for if it could be done it would have been done already, and to think of it has any government's political system ever worked from since the conception of id, that we can be governed by moral laws, that restricts the creative freedoms of a people to create in the image of creation, as a mother and father creates a life, a new born child, a miracle of nature, in their own image.

If I Am Then I Must Be

And so instead speaking of procrastinations of all sorts, even to his wife and children, and because my family were entrenched up to their necks in this oasis of triads of religious traditions, 'a set of threes a musical chord consisting of threes, a tonic, a third and a fifth now known as the us military strategic missile force made of flying mechanical birds, that flies, land based mechanical animals that run, as the human version of the wind in full motion, and underwater metallic fishes, as they form,' and so they could not understand, this kind of abuse.

So I did not get the help I needed, which led to me developing an alto ego, like the mild mannered Clark Kent, it is called a severe mental health problem, that was, that I resisted the hypnotic effects trying to control my life. And that was an idealistic thought from an ideology of funny ideas that I am a broken child, growing into manhood, that I must fit into the worship of those who have been abused, as children must do to appease their Gods of their own irrationalities of thought, sound, sight, smell, taste, and touch of that horrendous sexual act called sodomy, first practiced in Sodom and Gomorrah committed almost 30 years ago, is real in terms, and has a bearing on my life, as I walk the path to nowhere, like everyone else in life, that did not come back from that dead end road to perdition, and so later on in my life. I became a paranoid schizophrenic, and then even later I developed severe depression, and hearing voices, that were telling me that I am Hitler reborn, and then even later on, seeing things that were not there.

My main problem was my relationship with my father but unlike Hitler I did not see my father in those I hated, and thus tried to destroy my perceptions of who I thought my father was in me, by eradicating him from my memory, by trying to exterminate all life forms, that reflected him on the road going down a road called going nowhere. As Hitler riddle with guilt, as he blamed himself for the early death of his father, as I would have, as I put myself in his shoes, and imagine with empathy, how a tyrant would act, and by not obeying his father's wishes, and going to civil servant school, and so in his little id he went to, 'The War of The Worlds,' to prove to his dead father in the superstitious tradition of trying to appease the dead, as my ancestors from Africa were appeased in the worshipping of idols from generation to generation, that are made up pieces of wood to resemble the dead, it is called witchcraft, and like me Hitler consumed himself within his art in his school days, where fantasies become reality, indulging in his fantasies, as I did mines, just as I engulfed myself in my arts, trying to convince myself that one day I will be famous, when in truth I just could not express myself in words, so I learnt to speak my feelings by seeing and creating what I thought I saw on paper at that impressionable age of innocents, when eternity is shaped by an ideal, and when the world adored a ten year old boy who is no more, as I looked back in adulthood wondering where are my admirers now, where have they all gone, the one who said I had a baby face, the other one who said I looked so pretty in my school uniform.

I could not spell or write, but also, I was only ten, and I had never experienced life the way I have now, so I really had nothing to write about, except about what a normal ten year old boy would write about, and that I was the hero in love with my heroine, as I journeyed to save her from the Beast, who held her captive in his magical castle, far, far away in a land of dreams, and woes, and as Hitler failed, as an artist, so did I even though I was very talented, and won many awards for my artwork, I never graduated from art school instead I spent over thirty thousand British pounds taking out loans and getting grants, working day and night to gain what I thought was the way off the road called going nowhere, and in the end I ended at the end of the street called going nowhere, just like Hitler but however, he incensed his father when he told him that instead of following his father's ego, and joining the civil service, he was going to be an artist, which soured the father and son bond between them, and as his father grieved for his son he ceased to be anymore dying from a probable broken heart, as a man of pride humbled by his own image, his creation of his little id, which grew up to be known as the Frankenstein monster, the father of the modern day Homo sapiens, and with my father he told me at the age of about thirteen, that if I was gay, that he did not want anything to do with me but I was not gay, because like Alois Hitler who died 1903, Hitler's father, he was too a man of pride and ego, but unlike Hitler' parents he never married my mother, and never gave her a penny to support me, and so I grew up in abject poverty, whereas when Hitler was thirteen his father died.
His death did not cause his family financial hardships. Like my

irresponsible father, who could not keep his trouser zip, zipped up but that is the age-old story of human passion, and lusting after flesh, that is repeated in every generation, that has ever lived on this planet. And so Hitler's family had their own home and wealth whereas I had nothing. I started with nothing but a smile, as I entered mines. This was brought to light in my counseling of thought, touch, sound, smell and taste, that had in I think it was 2002. My counselor, which is called experiences, who was also on this same road, that leads nowhere, thought that I was focusing on nothing too much and not enough on something other than nothing, which makes no logical sense at all, which is very understandable but if I see my reflection' creation in nature, such as the rain, birds, and things like the earth in its natural form. I am sure you can understand why I was pre-occupied with nothing it is called a state of serenity.

Chapter 2

"This is my spiritual journey of the ethics of humanity, and not an ethereal one for the flesh and souls, the intellectual of the entirety of the human experience in flesh." The capacity of man to make decisions based on the animalistic nature that lies within us all. Hidden from the visible eyes, where they are vulnerable, naked, and ashamed, and hidden deep within the psychic personality, that turns into the psychotic episode of the existence in this modern world of machinery, metal and plastic, and greed. It is called economic growth. The grown child of the industrial revolution, as it silently cries out in its pride, and ego, as it arrogantly whispers, as a silent echo from a foreign land, 'only the fittest of the jungle survives,' like the Tarzan mentality that fictional character created by Edgar Rice Burroughs of the early 20th century's white heroic male complex. A strong man with rugged appearance and very muscular, the orphaned character raised in the jungle by apes. Now which you see portrayed in so many Hollywood's remakes of the Superman complex male, as the Godlike savior of the world, blowing it up over and over until the fabric of the universe screams out in pain and yells no more. Then begins to fights back in the form of global warming, and in the process killing, as many, as she can in the pursuit to bring order, and peace in her mechanistic skin uniform of pride, and ego, that she thinks she is right, and everyone else is wrong.

Then as I broke the psychic link between me and my dead father, so that I did not live his life or that he would not control me from the grave I composed my very own Epitaph, so that I can have peace with what he did in one moment of lustful passion, that brought me into being. For father I already know, what am I in your presence but a filthy rag, a stain on the conscience of heaven, for was not earth and heavens created through His mind? Then what do the heavens, the stars, the earth, rain, sun really think of me? They hate me. They know that I am just a vain insult in their presence. If it was not so then if I stay out in the sun too long will I not burn to death through cancer? Yes, Saturn has a part to do with it. If I go to the North Pole, will I not freeze to death? If I walk into the sea, will I not drown? If I jump off a mountain, will I not die in a horrible

If I Am Then I Must Be

death? Then I ask you what good am I to you father? Because you see not nor do, you acknowledge me. You say that the world was created for me, but if it rises up in anger against my crimes and that was to be born to a man like you in his hot lustful passion of the moment and to pollute it with my sins against its glorious heavens would I not die in a horrible and terrible death. Then what am I really to you father? What am I? I have no favor in this world to your deep blue sky, that now burn me to death with skin cancer. Instead, the sun retreats into the night deep black skies of the country. It neither sees me nor knows me then I ask you what am I in your presence but your shame. Then father why will not you let me die, and disappear into the clouds of nothing where my torment can begin. Where I know what I suspect.

Now that there is no hope for one such as me, if so ,where am I to go oh mighty father from your anger at what you as a human being did by creating me without a hope, and when we blow the earth up with bombs day and night in our playground of toy soldiers? Because you were never there for me what will, you call me. For 32 years it has been the same, just a vain memory in the corridors of time. Now do you understand why it is easier to make the decision to burn in hell of my conscience, for eternity, thus breaking the psychic link between me and you father? Because I know now I am made a prisoner of my conscience. I have no favor with man nor with you father, it is time to die. Why do you make it so difficult, because why should I come to your heaven? Then what chance do I really have? The truth is none. But a fading memory waiting to end for there is no hope for me. For I know what I really am in your presence oh father your mistake of a one nightstand. Oh earth, did you take pity on my sins and give me an education? Did you take pity on me and give a companion through my sufferings? Then what good is life to me now? What good is your goodness to me now father, now that you are dead, and in the grave to be remembered no more? Don't you understand I am but a vain memory to time, that time is running out, and I draw more closer to my descent into hell? Oh earth can't you hear death and hell calling me to come. "It is almost time," they say. Then why are you silent? Yes, it was my choice, but what choice did I have? Were you a real father to me oh dead man in the grave of forgetfulness? Am I not afraid of death?

Then how could I live? And now you answer me from beyond the grave in dark speeches, which I neither know nor understand. I ask you to show me the light, and you are silent. Why do you hate me so oh father? I cannot repent anymore. If you want my flesh or if I knew you would accept it as a sacrifice for my sins for killing your hopes of a life without taking care of your responsibilities, which you never did I would gladly give it and walk among the people of the earth, as a freak of nature but you do not accept sacrifices only obedience but if you are silent to me how do I know that I am being obedient? Why do you prepare my descent into hell oh heavens? Did not Jesus die in my place to spare me from it? Then why must I go there? Oh father you say no it is not so then answer this question. You say that faith is an act.

Then why do you act to give me a pound to feed the poor and myself, but you give your new wife and family, that are not even your own flesh, and blood good jobs, homes, partners, good cars, and honor, that they abused? Then what is my crime? Then what good is life to me now. My best years gone and they will never return. And I know that I am cursed, because I do not have that kind of favor with you oh dead father, I look around in your world, and I see nothing that I want, then why do you torment me oh father from beyond the grave? Is it my blood you want I would gladly give it? But you are silent towards me nor do you speak to me, as a son of yours for was I not made from your dirt? But as a dog without a master and you never once encouraged me, when you was alive nor did you change your anger towards me, so I suffer in silence, because there is none greater than you, and you are just in the torment, and punishment that you have cursed me with. I cannot argue my case with you because you are right.

I am but filth in your presence. You made me with your folly and you have put me to shame with that same wisdom. And all my tears are just but a vain memory in your sight, because they cannot change you, because you are right in what you did in your own eyes in this world. What chances have I against a man who could not constrain his lust for the flesh of the eyes? What hope do I have that you will be merciful to me, and have pity on me? The question is why would you? I cry night, I cry day but you are silent, in the night I am tormented by the darkness of your words, because I have not

If I Am Then I Must Be

found favor in the day. I am confused, because I cannot hear, because you do not speak to me in words I can understand. I believe I could except my fate, which is hell, if I understood why you have rejected me in your sore displeasure, at least have pity on me, and tell me why I have been punished for 32 years of my life? Why is my life in vain, and most important, why must I experience hell? In this way, my sentence is much more bearable when I am cast into hell. I can tell the dammed that you were merciful to me and told me why I am cursed and dammed forever. And as I composed my Epitaph to go on my tomb stone the universe cries and weeps for it knows that its sentence is just.

Chapter 3

But now known as the typical adventure movie that we all escape to, at one point or another, to fantasize about. It is now called escapism. But however, in truth it is running away from the truth of our reality in this modern world, which is based on economic progress, as we all know as capitalism without representation. Briefly just making money, more commonly known as greed. Now psychologist who works in cognitive recovery programs calls this kind of person psychotic, because this person believes, that the whole world is wrong, and that he is right, and is willing to kill, and murder anyone, and everyone who disagrees with his view of life. Hence, you could even call this kind of personality a severe paranoid schizophrenic, having a very bad hair day. Like the great John Wayne being immortalized, as the heart of what a hero is, in the hearts of many who live in the world, and now one of his prodigies, the remake of the John Wayne heroic hero complex, Batman Returns, our cape crusader trying to bring justice to Bat City, "If you devote yourself to an ideal you become more than a man." It is their philosophy.

Then Bruce Wayne asked himself, after he says you become something else he said, which is and as he answered, "A legend." And so we connect the dots with the legends of pop, the stars of rock, and roll who have brought the multitudes of souls from many generation to generation to worship on the road called going nowhere, and then to the new version of legend the feature film with Will Smith called, 'I Am legend.' where New York is wiped out in war of the intellects, and so New York is a nuclear war zone of ideological fantasies, that makes commerce, and so this is his legend for New York. And so Bruce Wayne can never get justice, because it is an illusion for him, because those who he seeks justice for are dead.

His parents, it is the guilt, that drives him on in his costume, trying to make the world a right place, to limit the fear of the others; "you must first master your own." Again their intended target is Bat city for their plan of mass destruction, it is the same as New York or what looks like New York, and so we have found the intent I believe

If I Am Then I Must Be

behind his words and after his parent are killed, and he lays on the floor in the hall of, 'The League of Shadows,' he drifts back to the event then he is seeing with his mentor's eyes, when he said do you still feel guilt for your parent's death? Bruce Wayne said, "My anger outweighs my guilt." And so we see on film played back to us in the Hollywood adventure film Batman with Christian Bale, as the wounded ego of the Homo sapiens, also the hidden conscience of Hitler's battle with his own guilt, that he felt at the age of thirteen, as he thought, that he was responsible for his father's death, by not going to civil servant school. "You must confront your anger," that is what I did for roughly 30 years of solitude, as I began to reconstruct my life, not based on living for the wound of sexual penetration but instead, healing the wound of sexual penetration, and so in the process becoming me, and not another version of Batman or Hitler, for that matter. And so witchcraft is no longer blinding the mind of my perception of humanity, the face that I see in my mirror of perception, reflected back at me, echoing my name, which is leading me to many needlessly deaths, and my rebirths, like the golden Phoenix, as I am reborn again, and again most just call it reinventing yourself but I like to be spiritual about these ideas of mines. And so training means nothing without the will or desire to act on what we learn, and if we do not know what the past is, and where it is leading us to, then how do we bury it, and live for today.

We take a part of this legend, that is put in boundaries, because of their attitudes, the middle wall of partition, that is being rebuilt by the want a be hero of our generation, who have sold their souls to the image of the image of the Beast, in the pursuit of the old age battle of gaining power to defeat our enemies, hence ourselves, which is a reflection of what we think intuitively about ourselves, triggered by those who we do not like for the ideal of fame, and power but by being segregated, and not being uniformed or being in unity to the naturally hidden eyes of self perception, in the invisible it is working in harmony for those who can see the unity, and where it lies Then the journey to life's meaning becomes a sign post, that in each generation, and those who can read sign languages can read the signs as *it* reflect them.

And so Bat city *is* styled on the phonetic sound of the word Goth, somebody who is considered to be uncivilized or even Goth music style, a style of popular music that combines elements of heavy metal with punk. As so many have tried, and failed, because they have missed the point of our existence, and that is not about economic growth without moral representation, or in a nut shell building without a conscience, like how the white western world has for many centuries robbed, enslaved the weaker members of our great civilizations, and ancient peoples, and murdered them to build what now is know, as the modern world. Making laws, that robbed the world's great ancient people of their dignity, as they lived, as one with the land, and each other, as a spiritual people.

You could just imagine, as you look around at the great cities of the world, especially from the old world how many poor, and innocent people died in misery in the pursuit of just plain old survival, and trying to live honestly before God, and man, building these great monarchal monuments to our great curiosity to delve into our alter egos, that we are a race of Superman moral men with extraordinary powers, like the mild manner Clark Kent, and his alter ego Superman. Or more to the point, economic progression towards our own ends, which eventually will lead to our destruction. Frankly, it is called protectionism. We all practice it. But however, it was meant to be a journey of a inner perception, that is still changing our reality, by changing our perception to line up with the individual conscience in us, to fit into a whole unit, and not to be conformed to one image, that is my image over all other images of mankind, which is the heart of all forms of racism, bigotry or more bluntly humanism in the form of socialism, were the people are considered one, and not individuals in a whole unit of different creative expressions. 'We the people, One nation under God, we will build a super race immune to the weaknesses of the Jews,' the mentally deformed, as we saw and our for-fathers experienced, mostly in World War II fight to destroy, and stop from entering our world but really started with Lucifer, when he wanted to make himself, as the same as God, and so on.' But that is like the same old story being rerun, as we get our daily dose of this character in our Hollywood fantasy flicks.

The great speeches of so many nations to produce converts, and disciples to their cause of nationalism, a desire for political independence, the desire to achieve independence, especially by a country under foreign control or by a people with a separate identity, and culture but no state of their own. A patriotic move by a proud, and devotion to a nation's cause, no matter the cost, even to sacrifice their lives for a dream that they would never ever see.

Even an excessive devotion to a nation or, as I would put it, a cause, that can never be achieved, such as terrorism or imperialism, or socialism, or democracy, even communism, a fanatical devotion to one's nation, and its interests, no matter how evil they are, which is often associated with a belief, that one country is superior to all others? Against a statement, that I have summed up in my foolish cynical look at humanity, I am a free man, not a slave to the desires of the few politicians who make laws to restrict our free and moral right to coexist with our fellow brothers who are of a different race, and colour, as with Noah after the flood he had three sons who are the founding fathers of all these nations but I was born free, and I will die a free man but in most cases those who believe in this statement, and are willing to fight for it usually die young. Is not this how Lucifer fell from his position in the kingdom of God? Is this not how Hitler fell when he lost World War II, is this not how the Americans were defeated in Vietnam? To encourage, and inspire many for what reasons other than to build great nations of superior intelligence, akin to the concept of Supermen with the ability to evolve into a super race of morally perfect beings. Almost Godlike if you think on it for a while. And the weaker element, such as in Nazi Germany, are eliminated by a process of mandatory murder, as in euthanize the weak, which we see in all forms now, hence the common one if I will not have anything to do with the gay community or he is too poor to be my friend. As in Nazi Germany in 1933, where those who were suffering from hereditary diseases were mandatory sterilized, in a Law for the Prevention of the Hereditarily Diseased by 1941, an approximately 72,000 people were murdered in this horrid way.

Now due to freedoms we have enjoyed for so long, we can now, in most countries, buy by law the information packs, that shows us how to take our own lives in a self suicide bid, to clean up our humanistic views, that only the strongest will survive, which is the main ethos in Nazism, and socialism, which is Nazism, and Communism, and also in some areas of democracy. If only the world knew and understood, they are the spiritual children of Hitlerism, and his concept of the Superman syndrome, the Third Reich, the Aryan nation or more bluntly, as we see it in the west, the hero complex, "the perfect man who is a good person a moral character, an exceptional man, a man possessing exceptional or superhuman strength, abilities or powers. Nietzsche's ideal man, according to the philosophy of Nietzsche, an ideal man who through creativity, and integrity is able to transcend good, and evil, and is the goal of human evolution," which is a concept of Darwinism or is what those who practice the Darwin religion are trying to get to, and it is a religion, because a religion does not allow the individual to be free of any concepts other than what is laid down by their founding fathers, and if you look at Jesus Christ, who came to change this concept, that mankind should serve one man's dream but instead have a relationship with a heavenly Father, as his own children, and to image, that the comic book hero Superman is based on the concept of evolution. A concept from the heart, and mind of Darwin, a scientist, and is found in the heart of civilizations, that prides themselves on being democracies. But yet all their laws are made to restrict the moral right of an individual to create in his own image something, that is good, and pure, as with the commands given to Adam and Eve in the, 'Garden of Eden.'

This Superman always doing right, and saving the world by killing his enemies, those who were different from him, this was the aims of Hitler who I know took the concept, that only the strongest, and pure German blood has the right to live, and all others must be eradicated from existence, like what Xexeres said to Leonidas, in the movie, '300,' from Darwin's theory the process of natural selection, instead of putting down his weapons of war, and sitting down at the table of debate, and discussing his differences with his enemies. The Superman, and in modern culture Superman has become the hero of many in the west, a comic strip created by a US writer named Jerry Siegal, and drawn by US artist Joseph Shuster, which first appeared in 1938.

"The alter ego of mild-mannered reporter Clark Kent, Superman is an almost invincible, crime-fighting superhero in a red cape, who was originally sent to Earth, as a child from the doomed planet Krypton. This story has been made into radio shows, musicals, television series, and feature films." " That is true, it also seems that the alter ego of Clark Kent can be traced back to the British story of the alter ego of the British mad men but even darker elements is the fact that Hitler also had an alter ego, as he planned his way of becoming the head of the Nazi party in Germany, as do so many others in general." Many believe that division is the real core element of racism, and in a sense it is from a certain point of view but however, it is the effect, that is division of trying to be a unit without considering where you came from, and not living who you are, with the governmental laws, both earthly, and heavenly to guide you in your creation in the image of God, Jehovah. Laws should be made to constraint evil men from hindering, and destroying the good in others. Not to protect the rich, and the immoral, because they can add great wealth to our nations is not this is the reason why the German businessmen wanted Hitler to be their chancellor? As we see in most countries and political systems of our day.

Chapter 4

It is once in a lifetime, that we as human beings have the chance to awaken from the river of sleep that everyone journeys along, until we reach death. As we enter into the river to Hades that is known in Greek mythology, and it could be the reason why many do not wish to even entertain the thought of where we go after we die. But however, it is once in many generations, that many nations have the chance to awaken, and change the destiny of a people. Many have tried like Martin Luther King Jr., who brought to the conscience of man, the notion of not to be judged by the colour of our skin but by the content of our conduct and our character, and through his conduct to awaken all America, and maybe even the world to the horrors of what we have become in our own eyes reflected in those we hate on the inside, he lived such a life of learning to love what he hated about himself in others, and so by doing so, he changed the conscience of many people, and so humanity moved one step closer to the great awakening of thoughts, ideas and ideals.

In other words, his conduct of character was his life, despite all the rumors we hear about his conduct. But he changed the ethos of the government in America, and the moral conscience of a nation, that has inspired many to dream, and just to live, as freemen, as we see with the first black president of the United States of America, not to see skin colour but to see beyond skin colour to the content of one's own character, and because Martin Luther King Jr., paid the price, many are no longer judged by the colour of their skin but by the content of their character. If we look at another great awakening but this in the Soviet Union, our enemies of the free world, because of their ideology, based on this false, awaken, when Lenin came up with the concept of socialism. Hence, without God, hence without a conscience, as we see how Stalin killed so many in his work camps, and for the people the same ethos behind humanism. However, at the beginning of humanism with Charles Darwin, you still pledge your allegiance to king and country. But Lenin had a greater idea but at the wrong time, and the wrong cause, because any government that does not take into consideration what Christ did on the cross of Calvary cannot govern its people in fairness, and truth, as we see in the historical history of just Stalin alone. Even though with some European countries they murdered, and robbed the innocent, and the poor in the name of Christ but as a doctor who is not trained by the law of the medical profession is not allowed to practice in the medical profession. It is the same with the law of Christ, if Christ did not murder anyone to get his message of a new creation in him by giving his life instead of taking anyone's life. And he showed us how he related to a Father, and not a God, as you see with many religions. So as the Darwin gurus would say, as with their campaign on the British Red Buses most recently, that there is no God so enjoy your life. They have a point, because the only thing that history has shown us of those who serve a God, is killing, mental slavery, and great poverty and misery.

That is why I believe that the God who Christ came to the world to reveal as a Father was so hard for the world to accept, even the Jews of that day. Because as the God of the Old Testament set up the, 'Law of Moses,' it was in my opinion set up to show, that you can never adequately serve a God by laws, because laws only reveals the mechanical side of a deity's nature. Laws only reveals the unemotional, and dead side of the nature of a God but however obeying a father's will, because you love him shows the human side of a God, the caring side of a God, and most important, the forgiving, and understanding side of a God, who is now a Father, and his love for his children, and all life, as you see many governments are trying to do with disastrous consequences, as we now see with this worldwide recession. Because a relationship to a God is a service based on a piece of paper, that is given to the people, as a law, when however, having a relationship with a father is about developing his nature, and learning how to love, and be compassionate to all life like he is to all life himself, and to care for the weak, and to correct the strong. Then those who professed to be his followers would also have the same conduct. So in a sense, all those who said they were Christ like, and killed others, to build their doctrine, like the Catholic church in the reformation period are not, by the law Christ laid down, and that was on the cross, he cried out to his, and our Father saying , "Father, forgive them for they know not what they do." Because the atmosphere was not conducive to change, and so evil and murderous men took hold of his concept of freedom, and used it to create communism, and other more vile forms of rule, that many good people died in, if we look at Abraham

Lincoln who is another great American, that had awaken to the ethos of what makes America so great, and that is it to promotes life, and liberty, and freedom. The chance to come to, and build the dream of the founding fathers, and to me in my interpretation is to be free to live in a country where politicians, and government is set up to enhance the people's movement to a free society free from poverty, turmoil, and control by a state government, that boast of freedom for the people but in truth are making laws to control their common people, like my government the British government. In other words a government set up to govern, just men, and just women, and to punish those who try to block the freedoms of the weak, to deliver the afflicted from harm to feed the poor, and to sacrifice their lives, when the ethos of their country, America calls, and that ethos is liberty. But as I have, leant liberty comes with a great price, and that price is the shed blood of our young, mostly our male voices, as they die on foreign soil for the liberty they so freely enjoyed back home in the land of the brave and the free. This is what makes America so great, and why I believe, that America is so hated throughout the known world, and why terrorist wish to blow up America. My idea of America is the last defense of liberty, and freedom for all both black, white, yellow, brown, all nations, creeds and colours, and sexual genders, as we see with the statue of liberty.

Chapter 5

As I watched, the stars fan the flames of their favorite music, the constellations of the Equatorial Zone, the constellations of the South Hemisphere, the constellations of the Northern Hemisphere, stars of different magnitudes. Making music but music that can be seen visually, far, far away, and not heard, unless you begin to imagine the heavens coming alive in the heart of your imagination. And in your imagination is the door to a new and undiscovered universe. It is called the universe of your heart, your spirit man, where all the treasures of God are found. It is where life started. For out of a sexual union of a passionate embrace is formed in the womb of a wife, a small life form, that grows for nine months, hidden from sight of man's eyes.

Then in an instance, a child is born, created within, where no one sees but God. It is where dreams are found, and not made, and come true, because those dream, found in your heart are built on a solid foundation, that is your Christ' conscious, if you choose him, and not the established church, which only condemns you for what they do in the dark. Not like the fantasies that you find in universities that only want to build the old system, a system of Egyptian commerce. The kind that leads a whole nation into slavery, those of the Israelites and the truth is they never left Egypt, and their slave masters, because the world is Egypt or based on its principals. And that is the humanistic thought pattern from the mind of a man who thought without the spiritual foundations of the thought realm, and that is conscience. Conscience is to look into the future at what effects your thinking, will take when you reveal it to the world. Hence, when Einstein first created the seed that now has created the nuclear weapon; did he know that the bomb would be used in Japan to stop World War II? Or did he ever think that Iran would want nuclear energy that may lead to them making their first atomic weapon? As the world uses Israel to build their towers of Babel, and then when they have the tower to their egos, they drive the Israeli out of their lands.

This has been happening for centuries. And now, that Israel has figured out the game, and had set up their fortresses, against the enemies of the poor, the rest of the capitalist and socialist world, where they can build their Promised Land, to serve their God Jehovah. And all these schemes come out of the west's heart but however, not America for America stands for freedom and liberty. In fact, it seems that slavery has never ended in the west, it is more complicated now but the west still wants to control the universe under the false pretense of democracy. The, 'Article of Independence,' the spiritual Africans were still slaves, and not considered human beings, and the black Nubian African Goddess was considered the white man's whore, his sexual conquest, in his attempt to be a man. So the very foundational of western democracy for the Afro American is founded on slavery, and racism, which came to a head in the days of Martin Luther King Jr.

Who made a statement, that he had a dream, that one day the Spiritual Afro American would be judged by the content of their character, and that is to love their wives as Christ has loved the church, and to live honestly and in peace working hard to produce to give to the nations, that they were sold into by slavery for a piece of dirt, that God has now given them for free but were denied by the animalistic behaviours of a few, in the sense of taking what is spiritual pure and turning them like spiritual vampires, draining the virtuous life from them, who corrupted their virtues, and turned a once proud nation into whores, and thieves to fulfill their humanistic pleasures of microorganisms evolving into animals, who evolved into the WASP's sexual desires, when in truth democracy does not exist in the west it is exist in the heart of every individual. If we look at the Western Europe at the time of slavery in 1789, Olaudah Equiano publishes his memoir. It is called, 'The Interesting Narrative of the life of Olaudah Equiano, or Gustavus Vassa, the African.' In his memoirs it contains the account of the, 'Middle Passage,' the African to American leg of the, 'triangular trade route,' and what made this account so unique was that it was from a slave's point of view. Olaudah's account of the shrieks of the women, and the groans of the dying rendered the whole, a scene of horror that was almost inconceivable. *'Taken from Channel-4 History- Britain Slave Trade, Website.'*

But yet still the best, that the west can do is to consider canceling the debts of these poor African countries, that their Egyptian type commerce made poor and caused these once great African nations to regress into war, corruption, disease, famine and chaos. There is hardly any mention of the governments of the west humbly confessing that they are canceling the debts of these African countries out of the remorsefulness of what their ancestors did to a once proud people. And to argue and debate in the houses of Parliament, whether or not to abolish slavery is hard to accept, because it shows that not all life was sacred, and that our British ancestors practiced the most horrid kind of racism, that has ever existed. A kind that murdered so many, and caused so much suffering, which still is felt today in both European and African societies. In 1780, the Quakers presented a petition to Parliament against the slave trade but it was not until 1863 that slavery was officially abolished in both the Americas and Europe.

That is a period of 83 years that it took the ancestors of the free world, and what we call the more humane, and modern world to end the most horrid kind of slavery that has ever existed. And the reasons why I think it took so long was that these nations of humanist were not accountable to higher power, their own conscience. And there were no other nations strong enough to take on the might of the Western and European governments. So the weaker nations were murdered, and mercilessly destroyed for a concept found only in Egyptian commerce, and that is greed, that dirt, and wealth is more important than the precious life, that God created in the, 'Garden of Eden,' to be celebrated on the earth in the years of life and freedom, to grow up without another race trying to tell you from their perspective what you are, what colour you are, because they want to label you, as a specimen, so that you can be controlled, as an experiment, in the thought process of changing what cannot be changed, the human heart.

And that is why through Christ's death, and resurrection, he created a new heart in a new man, the image of Christ in man, that has struggled against the society of man, that did, and does not want to change from their deprave lifestyles. As we see throughout history of how the weaker elements of our societies has paid the price of this great experiment, that Charles Darwin opened in his Pandora's box, that we evolved from monkeys, and that we are not accountable to our own conscience for what we do to each other.

Go back to Vietnam, how many young black men where given the freedom not to go to War, not many. It was the white middle class who were in college, that were spared the horrors set out by the western civilization for the poor, the weak and those who do not have a voice in politics. But if we look at the Jews, and their religion, they have tried to be true the original command given to Adam, 'Be Fruitful And Multiply And Replenish The Earth,' which the WASP has destroyed by killing them after they have built their commerce like Hitler and Stalin, Even the British kings and queens, and the worst, the church, down through to the ages, by developing the treasures in their hearts, and they have been successful, it is the thieves, and just pure trash who have deceived the Jews into building the world's economic system then they have killed, and murdered the Jews for centuries thinking that God of the Jews has not seen what they tried to hide in secret. It is true, that the Jews have developed a higher consciousness higher than the intelligence of the western nations, which can only rely on their education, that makes everyone like each other and not individual, so that the leaders can come up with gimmicks to fool the people, that their ways are the best.

However, as we now see it is all falling apart since the Jews left the world, and went into their fortress, away from the lies of the western civilization. It is like the black race, the white race took the Africans from Africa, and made them their whores and work slaves, and then they bred their women like whores, having their white wives, and their black whores on the side. Then when the civil rights movement came along, they gave them their rights but not a cut of the American dream, so the Black Afro Americans had to develop their own culture, language and music. Hence, they went inside into their universe to build from their treasures, what the white race could not do. This is what the Jews did for many centuries, the greatest example is what Hitler did to the Jews in Nazi Germany, having them build their commerce, and then blaming them for their ills. But one good thing it was the Christian nations, that died in battle leaving their lands, and homes to fight for the Jews, and liberty, while the rich hid in their fortresses, and the seed of the godly poor suffers, with high fuel bills, and having worked all their lives, and still have to pay into the system, that they sacrifice their lives for. In addition, we call this democracy, who said so? In fact, those leaders who promote this kind of governmental politics are no different from the Nazi, it is only that the name has changed but it is still the same system of the gas chambers, that Hitler killed so many undesirables.

In addition, the same experiments, that Hitler's scientist preformed on the weak, and vulnerable the British political system of humanism does with the seed, that shed their blood in the wars, that keep their dream of being worshipped, as Gods alive, by big class sizes, teaching their kids how to be whores by their sex education system in the schools. Not realizing, that it is their failed policies of their egos, that has caused the problems, in the first place, that British society now face, the drink problem, the smoking problem, the pregnancy problem, the gang violence problem. All began, because of government policies, by educated men of the Shakespeare era, a sodomite as well, as a well-known author so wonderfully quoted in his book on Shakespeare's life. You see the hidden secret of life is a people who hold the power, and make the laws control a nation, so they are to blame for all the ills in a nation. It is so simple but yet, because many are trying to be a have ago hero, they think in their arrogance, that they can change the heart when God said before he flooded, in Noah's day, the world with his tears of pain in the great flood, 'that the imagination of man is evil all he does all day is to think up evil and murder the innocent,' like in Iraq, Vietnam, Korea, Somalia, Ethiopia, Rwanda, Sudan, Bosnia, and many more. In addition, remember they are our brothers, and sisters, mothers and fathers, for all proceeded out of Eve's stomach, as we see from one generation to the next, in one family line, as all the children of that family comes out of the female of the species. However, all that is good in this world came out of the Jew's heart, out of their universe within them, and because they refused to bow to man's way, as we see with the ethos of the American Indian, and the underrepresented in this modern, and ancient world, when man made a promise of land to them, of freedom to roam on that land, they would break it when they found gold on it. In addition, because they had guns their law was the ultimate worship of the nature of Gods or dies a miserable death.

Chapter 6

I saw that my spiritual growth had begun to grow again. That is the ability to love myself for whom I am, and not what the world wants to see me as, I am able to look at myself in all life, and find truth of who I am, what I don't like in myself I will see in what I think, and say, as a correction for others, so by loving what I hate in others I am loving what I hate in myself.

Many years ago my growth had stopped, for I believed in the illusion of fantasies, that this visual music, that the stars creates, instead of going through the mirror into the reality, that would have led me to the truth of who I am and in man, a reflection of my family through many generations of life, from one parent to another, until I came out of my mother's loins in flesh made from the earth, and the life of God breathed into my nostrils, and so I become a living creative, being in the image of my ancestors, who were and are black Africans, and Asians from India, to reflect the divinity of my family in the earth. But the humanist who creates servitude, such as debt to enslave the poor of mind, and will with credit schemes, such as mortgages, so that they, the great hope can live as Gods, while we the poor are their servants fighting their wars and cleaning their wash-pots, while they experiment with our children, by feeding them lies, that we evolved from monkeys, and that we are not created in the image of our ancestors, to create in the earth from our ancestral like natures. Instead we are taught in schools about our past failures, and so nothing grows, and the human race can never reach enlightenment, and that is that Christ through our ancestors created a reflection of himself to be him in the earth, and Adam was meant to grow up from a child into the man of the reflection of God in mankind.

As I reflect on the creation of the galaxies, by intelligent design, and not as Steven Hawkins, and other mad scientists, believe, that the galaxies began with a big bang. This theory began with the ethos of Charles Darwin, and that we evolved from monkeys. Now to many it might not seem as much but to a spiritual man created in my ancestral tribal nature, that man can see the truth, as he looks back through history, or rather his story, the story of the WASP, who have killed, murdered, stole, raped, and simply destroyed all that is spiritual in other cultures, that were close to God in nature, so that they could build an empire of debauchery sex, wealth, and over indulgence. If we look at England, and how in the, 'Victorian Age,' they ruled the world with blood shed in the name of the Antichrist calling him Jesus Christ who never took a life, or stole someone else's property, and turned the whole human race into whores, thieves, murderers for greed, most commonly known as the Beast, as they acted like Beasts to steal, and to create in this century all the ills, that are seen in the third world. Because it was the Europeans colonialism, that created the world's political system, and that is based on Charles Darwin's theory of evolution, which simply means, that we are not accountable to a higher conscience, and that is life is worth more than a piece of mould, that most women of the western world wears on their bodies to look beautiful.

Now that scientists have found water on Mars, but for six thousand years, humankind, those who follow the intelligent design theory, knew from the book of Genesis, that God divided the waters in the heavens, and the waters in the earth. So if these scientists had any sense they could buy a copy of the bible, and read it for themselves. It would be far lest cheaper than what it cost to build a rocket to go to Mars to see if water was ever on that planet. Could you imagine how many hungry mouths in third world countries the money that it takes to send men into space, and put probes on the planet of war Mars in mythology, could feed? In addition, which would be more humane saving lives or seeing if life ever existed in space? Yet it is indicative of the nature of Darwin's philosophy, that the WASP has no conscience, as they cut up animals in experiments to make, 'make up,' for women, and other horrid experiments preformed on animals who cannot speak out for themselves, and is this what we call progress? Also scientist could also look at the DNA make up of the flesh of man and see from the bible, that we came from the dust of the ground, as written in the book of Genesis.

In addition, I would think that it would be very easy to see, that even without the bible or all the scientific tests, and money spent to do this kind of research by the fact that God said from dust you came from, and to dust you shall return. Yet scientist had to go to college, and spend over 40,000.00 pounds for a degree, and then the tax -

payers' money to do research, that commonsense would tell you, that it is so. It is kind of like Satan's logic gone to seed, that he can defeat the great Christ of God. When, as with all life, Christ created them, and so if he created the angels, and humankind, and he knows the future, would he not have made man, Satan, and his crowd to fail at their attempts to be intelligent? As the humanist, prove everyday of their lives, just like Charles Darwin's theory, that it just happened. As if a baby just appeared on the earth, feeding itself until it became an adult of the process of million of years. In addition, babies where having sex with other babies to bring more babies into the world. That would mean, that for million of years babies have been breaking British Law, that forbids sex under a certain age. Maybe that is why many children are becoming parents, like their ancestors.

However, the ideology, that we just happened, and we are not accountable to our own moral conscience has created so many wars, death, plagues, injustice, and social abuse in this last century alone. In addition, the educated establishment makes so much money from the misery that their ancestors have caused to build this great western world. In fact, if you are good at math go to a building, and try to compute how much innocent blood was shed for each brick, that is laid in that building our memorials to progression, as a more humane society, that is anyone we do not like we kill. Have you heard of the saying ignorance gone to seed? When we look at a decaying body buried for many years, how it turns back to dust but not the hair and the skeleton.

We can see that flesh is the same material, that the dust is made of, because if it were not the flesh of the dead body being dust it would not go back to the dust, as God commanded when man decided they wanted to be responsible for their own right and wrong, by eating of the tree of the knowledge of good and evil, and so also with being responsible for our right and wrongs but also paying the price for them too, that is the Lake Of Fire for eternity. Maybe it is the crucified flesh of the dead body of Christ on the cross. By somehow finding peace with this image of the Son of God, on that cross, that I had slain through becoming a sinner by disobeying the commandments to love and not to hate myself by hating others, especially my abusers those who turned me into a freak of nature but however, in time I learnt to forgive, and so I healed myself. The scientist such as Charles Darwin, I would have been reconciling myself to God, not through the churches, a man's doctrine-a man's interpretation of a holy man's love for all humankind but my own relationship with a holy God that I could cherish for eternity. I can now image in the body of flesh talking, and walking with the Son of God, in the earth, and stars, listening together to the heavenly orchestra, as we have relationship, supping tea - the British way of traditional life. Is this what the mad scientists like Steve Hawkins are trying to disprove, that we are sinners, and that the wages of sin is death. However, the gift of God is eternal life? And it is a free gift, that you do not have to pay anything for it just give him your sins, that is that you can make it on your own and take his right standing with a loving Father.

Chapter 7

Because I did not believe in the Hollywood fantasy, that the humanistic churches are portraying of him in Britain, and that God is an angry God. They tried to prove, that he was the God who was punishing me for killing his son on the cross but they have forgotten, that I met the real Christ, as a child, and he came into my heart to sup with me, and he has been there ever since the time of my youth. Therefore, when I look at the sunshine, as it goes down on a lazy summer's afternoon. I do not see an angry God, who is mad at the world, as the British churches are preaching from their pulpits. Nor do I see that all these great creations just happened for no reason at all. In our lives we make choices, nothing we do is by chance. All happens for a reason. So I could never believe in the lie that the scientist are portraying that life just happened. If that were true, then what hope would we have in the after life, when we leave this world? Where would we go? How would we separate those who have done great crimes against humankind from those who have helped humankind? You see, which generation would pay the full price that humanism has cost in the toll of lives taken, and the amount of bloodshed, that has occurred over these many centuries. In the cause to satisfy the satisfaction of some mad scientist, 'Jor El,' that life just happened, and that we are not accountable for the evil that we have done to each other. What logic is there in believing that life just happened?

I see a loving Father who wants to fellowship with all humankind in a loving way. Who wants to help humankind to find his son, and gain, through peaceful, means what they desire from him. In addition, all of a sudden it became so clear to me, that God is a loving God, and not an Olga, as we are taught to believe by the witches in the British churches. I also realized that I am an individual not a national insurance number, and certainly not a statistic in a report placed on some politician's desk, to prove that the government is working, when they are not. I am learning that I want to be an individual, like as a child free from the burdens of laws that restricts our creativity and heighten the governments' pen pushers in White Hall. It was the government, that made laws forcing us as children to be educated by the Beast, their system of education, because they had past laws that kept us working in work houses of the educational systems of this world, when we should be with our parents, as they taught us right and wrong, and how to love each other by loving ourselves. We would have grown into great godly men and women of this world. But the egos of the well informed in knowledge of the upper class desired to be worshipped as Gods so they purposely created an underclass of underachievers so that with all the facts they learnt about the past in European history they would capture the hearts of the poor, and make them worship them as Gods as we see in the, 'X Factor,' as many who are talented are forced to degrade themselves for a piece of a dream, that does not exist. After all, where are all those who lived on this earth a hundred years ago? They are in the grave to be only remembered as idols and false Gods, leading many away from the real God that lies within. In addition, it was only Christ as a true son of the only God that has power to raise the dead, as he proved when he raised Christ his firstborn son from the dead.

No other religion records, that their delegates sent by their God had the power to raise their delegates from the dead to prove that their delegate was in fact from a real God, and not an idol, created by man's curiosity. Therefore it is only Christ who has been victorious over the greatest enemy of humanity, and that is death. So it would be prudent to assume that Christ, and the gospels not the Old Testament holds the secrets to eternal life, and that is his words, that he spoke in Matthew, Mark, Luke and John should be taken very seriously but what do the historians try to prove, that he did not rise from the dead, and that he had sexual relations with the woman called Mary. The Christ God image, that will help the poor create their dreams, to live honestly, and not as whores for the educated, and the experiment of the Politicians outside of the ten commands, which God gave to the Israelites for all the families on the earth. The most important one of them all, 'Thou shalt not kill,' thy brother, thy sister, thy father, thy mother and thy children for greed, calling it progression, that we are bringing peace to the world, and think that God would not avenge the slain dead on the living.

In addition, these Social workers of government are not a profession in my view; yes, it is more of a vocation, based on the effects of human understanding without compassion. It proves nothing to be a

Politician, only that you are adept to the social ills in life. However, for me to study either music or languages, and so it will help me to learn how to communicate what is buried deep within me those treasures that God has placed in my heart for his kingdom, I am not saying that politics is a possessive field of an avenue to greatness but there is a difference between building the kingdom, and caring for the dying. From my perspective as a great skilful singer of language, my talents will bring me before great people to give my testimony as well as my language skill will bring me to the poorest of the poor. I am not a statistic in a scientific experiment that is controlled from White Hall by the pen pushers. I am a man born free that will die a free man.

I am skillful at a thing I know who you are, and who you are not. I must know my limitations, and where I can excel, my strengths, and weaknesses, and I must learn how to master them. Therefore, I must know how to speak in that language. I must know them to be understood, and I must know how not to be understood. Can Politicians create an environment where this can happen for the poor in spirit? Can universities of humanistic thought patterns create a learning environment that caters to the differences that promotes racial harmony, instead of just focusing on man's way of life? That is forgotten, after they robbed, murdered, and stole to build it. What good is there in reliving the past why not live for the present to build the future, instead teaching our children about the pass of another, an alien race that brought us here in slave ships? That fought the Chinese to keep the opium roots going, who build their slave labour in India, and much more.

The truth from my point of view is, if you are truly free from the prison, you will spend most of your time alone in solitude, as you reflect on why you were there in the first place, and also on what is the right course of action to take on your journey to somewhere, thus coming off the road going nowhere. To travel back along the road of pain, and endless regrets being directed by your guiding angels, back to the, 'Garden of Eden,' where you can eat from the tree of Life, that is partake of the true doctrine of Christ, that is to love all people, not just a special selected group, as those who say they belong to him do. In addition, on how you got out, did you go through the door or did you climb over the prison fence. In addition,

If I Am Then I Must Be

I am a merciful man, because it would take a lot to move me to say what I truly believe, and what I know as truth. It is like a fool who dreams up excuses why, to make good, ignoring the facts that smoking kills, just to enjoy his moment in time until reality sets in. He is about to die from his obsessions with a chemical fixation, and he spends the rest of his time warning others of something, he could not control himself, trying to make penitent for his perceived mistake. But not admitting deep down that it was his pride that he was always right, that killed him, by not admitting that he was vulnerable, a weak creature of habit, so his new habit in his arrogance is to tell about the dangers of smoking, to give him dignity in his death. And once your words dies so do you and they no longer are words of an individual but the words of one collective thought, in a sense a zombie with no conscience or ability to think outside what is presumed to be life, as we know it. Therefore, the words spoken shapes the intent of the heart, while the heart has begun changing the personally or the ethos of who that person is and why that person exist, and makes important the reason from within his conscience, as to why continue to live.

And to me an ambassador is, I would think, is a sates man who is sent by a king with the seal of a king's approval that is the cross of Christ into a foreign kingdom to mediate on behalf of the king, and enforce his decrees, and established based on the king's governmental practices his kingdom. Now an ambassador is a diplomat at such, and his first opinion is to look at the situation, as it is from his point of view the king, the kingdom and the kingdoms where his subjects are held captive, and then debate with the king on the best way forward, that is based on divine laws, which over rules any rights of the natural governments or any claim they may have with the citizens of that kingdom. In this case, all those who have no voice in government are the king's subjects. So it is not about being weak or fearful or even restricted by the by laws that hinders the king's decrees from coming to past, it is just being fair, just, and also in a gentlemen in nature knowing that if the king wishes he can forcefully push through his decrees.

Chapter 8

As I came back to normal thought and spent less of my time ruminating, I remembered Peter in Massachusetts, I remembered him as he steered at a woman's ass to his eyes, that had no shape, it was not a sexual object, but yet he seemed to be sexuality aroused by the idea of having sexual intimate union with her bottom. Nevertheless, the most amazing part is that he could not understand why I never felt the same way, he did.

He could not accept that I was not like him, which proved, that the only reason why he wanted to be friends with me was that he thought I was a reflection of his corrupt and lustful desires, which was not the case. He served Lachelle as her faithful servant driving her there, and here and everywhere, except to his bed, which was the point of being her driver, but I thought nothing of it at first until Lachelle sat down and told me her hidden story. Her inner pain, he only serves her as her faithful servant, hoping one day to join with her sexually. Nevertheless, what she could not understand, that she was also being deceptive in their union, because you could not really call it a friendship of sorts, because she was using him as her personal whore, as she was the pimp.

He was only there to provide a service, so she puts up with his player attitude, while he thinks he is making headways into her uncharted territory, hidden in her pants. So in me, she saw a soft cushion for her tormented conscience, because her struggles with the mother she hated, her moral statute as a devout woman who raised her kids in her image, and not in the children's image, and so they both rebelled against her moral traditions of that you must first love the man you marry. But Lachelle was marrying her man, because he was rich, and I would think that she should learn how to love him as she built her fantasy life to hide her pain, and hate for her mother for loving her for who Lachelle is, and needing to support her hypnotic theory of how a young child should grow up into adulthood. Her younger, the bucktooth saber lioness followed in her big sisters' footsteps she got engaged to a sailor who she never saw that often. Because he was always on his ship serving his country, instead of serving her, so their relationship was like a long distance call. A relationship of convenience whenever they saw each other, it was like calling a friend in China long distance. "How's the weather over there?" "Did you have anything nice to eat?" "Did you meet anyone of interest while at sea?" "What did you do while we were apart?" And so on, no one wants to evolve intimately by allowing themselves to be vulnerable, in this way they are building an ice fortress like the fortress of solitude Superman's thinking tank of ice. The middle of Antarctica where superman built his fortress of solitude to reflect on the potential that humanism has. However, their fortress of solitude is a fortress, and a prison of their conscience, the insane part that will drive them to insanity as they grow together, and to die alone. Is that they have built their relationship on their percepts, based on feelings, such as pride, jealousy, hate, arrogance, which are the seeds of humanism. Trying to protect their vulnerable natures, which is, 'I need you to love me for what I am and not what you are trying to create in me a reflection of you,' the heart of racism. Fantasy as I wonder while you make love to me as I open my eyes, and I see yours are still closed while your tongue is down my throat, and I am wondering why can't you look at them, but you can stick your tongue in my mouth, and give my teeth a cleaning after we have just had a Chinese take away, and I have eaten garlic are your eyes closed, because the taste of the garlic on your tongue, with my spit is making you sick or is it that you are ashamed of me, and I am only the woman that you can get to fulfill your sexual fantasy, and if I am who are you fantasying about that you are making love too?

Chapter 9

Homo sapiens being another variety of the modern human man, like the many different models of the old Ford automobile being made new and upgraded every so often, made for the consumer's needs, the only extant species of the different makes of the modern man from the archaic, and outdated specimen of the species of man, that also included other species named just as there were other brands of the old model Ford automobile. The Homo family Hominidae from modern Latin literally meaning wise man but in my eyes of a man living with schizophrenia I call it all knowing man always having the answers based on his own logic, and not based on the cosmic truths of the universe, that our great grand parents knew or more to the point, our great ancestors had discovered in ancient times.

The Homo family Hominidae from the Greek homos ultimately from an Indo-European word meaning one, which is also the ancestor of English. Homo Habilis the extinct ancestor of Homo sapiens, an extinct ancestor of the modern human being, living approximately 1.5 million years ago, and characterized by its ability to make, and use tools from modern Latin literally meaning skilful man. Homo erectus extinct ancestor of Homo sapiens, an extinct ancestor of the modern human being. Homo sapiens living approximately 1.5 million years ago, and known by fossils to have had an upright stature, a smallish brain, and a low forehead. From modern Latin literally upright man, and then the homoeroticism homosexual eroticism, that is focused on or inspired by people of the same sex the one thing all these models of the Homo sapiens model need to be the, 'New Age Man,' and to feel good about themselves.

The final version of the modern man the Homo sapiens, a perception of his own reflection, just as he looks into the mirror to groom his facial features, to shave his bread, to comb his hair and to put cream on his face, so that he is attractive to his prey, the Homo sapiens, a perception of his same reflection as in the mirror in the morning, and throughout the day as the mirror, that he perceives himself to be in life down through the corridors of time as he tells his story in the form of his history, which is his-story personified in oral, and

If I Am Then I Must Be

literary form, and not ours as he begins to label his experiences like in his own appearance, that he is trying to create each morning to show to the world, that he is Superman, and can save the day with his ego, and pride as he see that he is right, and all others are wrong. Therefore, individualism is born, the plastic smile of chaos. For one Homo sapiens sees differently from another Homo sapiens, and so there is no absolute truth in the world of make believe but a reflection of what we see in our mirrors of our past historical lives. As we try to build, an existence based on this word, 'If I am then I must be.'

Moreover, so to one Homo sapiens red is the colour of blue and to another Homo sapiens the colour red is as the colour black. Hence black the dark recesses of the human heart with all its skeletons in its black opaque closet, and the blue the sea of black emotions, that screams at us telling us, that we are growing old decaying as the old model Ford automobile wears out after so many miles of luscious usage. So we like the obsessive car owner spends all his free time working on his car, while his family grows hungry starved of the affection of this new Ford model man, the modern man we go under the knife to recoup, and remake the old model of the archaic man, the Hominidae Homo Habilis into a new kind of man part flesh, part dirt and part plastic. Like all the models of the Old T Ford, and new automobile needed to run, and operate in a modern world, and that is oil the black gold of our utopian eroticism of the sexual revolution, that has gripped humankind for decades. Since the first man said, 'If I am therefore I must be, and so he was.' And from the molecules of chemistry, the smallest of a chemical compound, the smallest physical unit of a substance, that can exist independently, consisting of one or more atoms held together by chemical forces, the smallest part of elemental portion into, which an element can be divided, and still retain its properties, made up of a dense, positively charged nucleus surrounded by a system of electrons, that divide into a chemical reaction for some removal, transfer, or the exchange of specific electron, that becomes the basic particle of dark matter, indestructible, and indivisible, first proposed by the ancient Greek philosophers as the fundamental component of the universe.

As all he thinks about is how sexy he looks to the opposite sex, and their companions, the same as they admire themselves in the mirror of life. The race of Supermen that came from the mind of the Nazi but existed before, in the Greeks, the Romans, the British Empire and so on as they tried to exterminate all other inferior races to create just one new race in the tradition of the ancient concept of the natural man The philosopher, a creature who studies life as an experiment, and it reality known as its perception in the mirror of life as in the reflection of a man's ego as he makes himself look pretty, and perky, the concept of being sexy in his own perception of his own reflection in this modern man, like as a couple buys a certain type of automobile for a specific purpose of their reflection from the mirror of life, which is their perception of the colour red, and so does this modern man creates an illusion of the word, 'If I am I must be,' and so spends his whole life trying to explain why he must be as the man who see red as an opaque black, and the man who sees blue as the volatile emotions, and they both seek to understand, and explain the nature of what they have perceived in the mirror of life as they think deeply, and seriously about their perceptions of life, until the day of manifestation of their creation.

When war breaks out, it is called science The Third Reich, the Aryan nation or more bluntly the word, 'If I am then I must be,' and another hero is born to wage war in the right of justice, thus denying all others justice, in the pursuit of the ultimate justice, and that is to eradicate all entities, that are of the old ways as all the old model of the Ford automobile are disposed of, because they are no longer relevant to today's world but yet Mr. Ford took the same car, and just made it differently to suit another generation, in the pursuit of the American dream just like how Hitler disposed of the Jewish people, and in so creating the their ultimate tomb, and that is for Israel so when he speaks from the grave his orders to destroy Israel they are destroyed as they are now in a life and death struggle in Israel.

The perfect reflection of the modern man the Homo sapiens male, who is a good person with a moral character, an exceptional man, with superhuman strength, abilities or powers, as Nietzsche speaks from the idea of his ideal man, in the modern man, according to the philosophy of Nietzsche, an ideal man who through creativity and integrity is able to transcend good and evil, and is the goal of human evolution for just a select few who uses his name, 'Karl El,' to condemn the world, by saying, because you do not think like us, or act like us you are immoral, and sinners, and you are damned for eternity. The core root of individualism or could it be elitism, which leads to separation but not in the sense of colour, creed, or race but in the sense, that you are not of a select group, which is the same ideals, the ethos called perception, 'If I am then I must be,' which still exist but in that case it is like a tradition, that have come back from the dead to claim its victims, those who follow the cultural aspects of perception, 'If I am then I must be.' Therefore, in the tradition of, 'If I am then I must be,' creates in the image of, 'If I am then I must be.'

Moreover, whatever was will be, and so they who follow this conception of the mind of the wise man or the philosopher will be what was and not what is, as many are trapped by this very cunning illusion. That is if you live in the past you will live the past, and it is predictable, the future of course, because it is the past relieved but with different names, and different perceptions. Just as the Old Ford automobile is continually remade to suit the consumer's fantasy of grandeur, the illusion of feeling, that one is great or grand, and very impressive as we are taught in the school of advertising, and thought but in reality it is the same old piece of junk, that makes Homo sapiens lazy with four wheels an engine, some metal, and other parts of inanimate particles, not active or lively but the thought of the perception of the beholder, the owner of this piece of a concept considered to be without life.

The Frankenstein monster reanimated to bring death and destruction as the drunken motorist kills another innocent life in the pursuit of the consumer's fantasy of grandeur, the illusion of feeling, that one is great or grand, and very impressive as we are taught in the school of advertising, and thought. "I believe I can fly, I believe I can touch the sky, I think about it every night, and day, Going through that open door" Red becomes a different kind of black, and red becomes a different kind of blue. Nevertheless, it is the same black, and the same blue. Is not that what Winston Churchill said when he led a small Christian nation like Britain to victory over the Nazi Empire? As he so boldly stated to know the future, you must know the past. In addition, you saw for yourselves the victory that was won for freedom, and liberty of those individuals who would lay down their lives for such a concept that never existed. For who told, them that they were not free to chose their own destiny. I did not. Nevertheless, did he ever consider that if you know the past you would only create the past in the future? In addition, as we are taught in primary school, 'one plus one will equal two,' all the time, and it will never change because it is predictable, and guaranteed. Therefore, by teaching the past we live the past, hence the ideal that, 'one plus one will always equal two,' and so life will always be predictable to the tyrant who wishes to rule the world. Like the famous concept of the Antichrist, or the Dictator, the imperialist or the Communist, maybe even the Socialist, the humanist, and of the course the democratic man. In addition, so with this growing recession, which is the past in the 1929s then, came war to claim the prize of those who lived in the past, and not in the present moment. Hence, like the Afro-Caribbean diet, which is made of high starch foods, and rich foods that in the days of slavery were prudent to consume, because of the amount of energy that was needed to do such hard work? Now they eat these kinds of foods simply, because they came from that cultural perception. So red becomes the opaque colour of black as the earth is put in the grave to be closed, and never open to the light of day again, the death of life, and so because the reason in the first place why they had to eat this high starch diet is no longer relevant they are dying in their numbers from all kinds of creations, that they created such as disease, high blood pressure, diabetes, and so on. 'For If I am then I must be,' then I am and so I have created in my own image of, 'I am then I must be.'

One sense of the word my destiny and that is the grave where the fruits and rewards of my perception of the colour red the disturbing opaque colour black where there is no light of day. No stars, no clouds, just opaque black the end of being. In addition, the emotionless blue. The natural colours of the rainbow, forever a fading memory of the natural colours of the creationistic, mysticism, the writing of fiction, poetry, or even drama are exercised as all are put into a position of being unable to understand or explain the mysteriously opaque black darkness, that is so hard to understand for there is nothing to see, nothing to perceive anymore for the light of the reflection of Homo sapiens is now extinguished by the sudden coming of the opaque black, the darkness, and so perception cannot be perceived in Polydemon, which awaits me, and where the wealthy make their abode. What good are money, riches, and fame in the darkness where no light is seen, and is never to be heard of again? Where reflection is no more so perception dies, and becomes an empty vast ocean of emotions in the deep blue sea of endless regret as the illusion of perception is finally realized. The words, "what did I live for?" For in the light of perception, as the rich ruler tormented by the opaque black, the darkness of his once dead soul now rotting, a rotting diseased corpse stands alone in the darkness as no light can be shed on his predicament as he looks on the light bearer Abraham the father of the Jews, and the gentile nations, those who saw in the light of truth. And obeyed as he said, ""I am the way, the truth and the life, no one come to the Father but through me and if you believe in me you shall walk in the light and never again walk in the darkness," of the reflection of perception in the mirror of belief in intuitive soulical revelation the belief that personal communication or union with the vague opaque black of the darkness of our souls and lustful desires is the way to enlightenment and liberation from the, 'Law of Creation,' as so many have tried to change through the mirror of perception by perceiving that they are and therefore must be like the murderer who is sentenced to death screaming in his heart unseen from the eyes of curiosity, "I do not want to die," but yet is powerless to stop his execution for it is the Law and the Law must be obeyed by everyone. As the rich ruler's corrupted, conscience begs for the light in the darkness so that perception in the mirror of understanding of self can once again be seen."

As the famous wise man, the son of God, and the son of man said, "what does it profit a man to gain the whole world, and loose his soul in the darkness of self, the land of Polydemon, where the emptiness, and endless regret, and the gnashing of teethe resides. What does it profit's the rich to enter the hot overwhelming oceans of Polydemon, never to return to the land of the living the land of light for Cerberus, the three headed dog who guarded the entrance to the underworld known as Hades will not let them leave this place of opaque black, and blue emotions where they are escorted by the boatman Charon, who would ferry them across the Styx but only those ghosts who could pay the fare would be allowed to go," and the fare is this as a young wise man once wrote "And this is the condemnation, that light is come into the world, and men loved darkness rather than light, because their deeds were evil. For every one that doeth evil hateh the light, neither cometh to the light, lest his deeds should be reproved." Therefore, those who could indulge in their reflection of lust, and decadence, their idealism that she is the chosen path answered, found when this truly wise man said. Then answered all the people, and said, "His blood be on us, and our children." And so Charon does as he did When Pilate saw that he could prevail nothing, but rather tumult was made, he took water, and washed his hands before the multitude, saying, "I am innocent of the blood of this just person: see ye to it."

If I Am Then I Must Be

Chapter 10

As soon as nobody with half of the end of functions of the central anxious system calculated by brainwave through the leisure interest on an electroencephalogram, over a set period of time, since its occurrence can allow the termination of the life support or the removal of organs for transmission to a new plantation of Homo sapiens as the modern man tries to go beyond an offensive term meaning of extremely low intellectual abilities, the anatomy of the appendage of thoughts of feelings, the controlling centre of the panicky system in versatility of the connection to the Darwinism, the tree of life, the spinal cord of the anatomy of the discord of harmony in the enclosed head of the philosopher's moral effects consisting of a mass of nerve tissue, and nerve supporting, and de-nourishing tissues, the centre of thoughts, and emotions, and regulates bodily activities, and unable to stop thinking about the questions that so allude the modern man, and so the brain of intellectual pursuit of the word being, becomes a beating heart in the violently turmoil of the intellect, nourishing the agonistic nature of the Homo sapiens, trying to affect evolution in an effect of appearing manufactured like the manufactured automobile as it is assembled on the assemble line of progression, into a better society of thought, 'If I am then I must be,' an exaggerated literary argumentative of the Renascence of Europe, that tends to argue, and is eager to win the argument of the tree of life, that just cannot exist in the absolute reality, made up of non realities, instead of the reflections of the perceptions, that we see in the mirrors of life. And Jesus the Lord God commanded conscious thought contained in the earth of creation, a part of a whole part, in one part, hence a conscious fraction contained in time for it was spoken, that time shall only be one hundred twenty years for thought, and that is to be that, 'which I think am, and then it will be no more,' but a fading memory, like the fading sunset as it fades into the winter night of stars, and bright clouds of the night's cosmos far, far away, like a dream, that when we wake up from in the bright morning of the light of our perception of our own reflection in the mirror of life, it is gone without a goodbye my sweet lullaby in the minds of the young, who are trying to save the world in the saying of the Nietzsche Superman, "of every tree of the garden thou mayest freely eat, but of the tree of the knowledge of good and evil, the thought, 'If I am then I must be,' thou shall not eat of it, for in the day that thou eatest thereof thou shall surely be, 'that which that is and no more,' and the fruits there of, you shall be, and so conscious thought contained in the container of the earth of creation did and from his loins came Homo sapiens, 'If I am then I must be,' to be no more," just a fading memory of the imagination of the race of Superman trying to bring peace to the world by creating wars, famines, starvation, disease, poverty, illness, servitude, slavery, decadence, crime, and all conscious thought contained in the containers of dust, for all think alike, a car is a car to the Chinese, the Indians, the Hispanics, the Americans, the Europeans, the Jews, the Arab and the American Indians, and in so all relative conceptual thoughts of every single nation on this earth have the same names for the same experience, that every single person on this earth encounters in their existence of touch, taste, see, smell and hear, consumed from the tree of knowledge of good and evil from their loins came Nazism, Hitler's philosophy as he saw in the light of perception, his own reflection, and so created himself by creating the Aryan race, The Third Reich, the Aryan nation or more bluntly as we see it in the heroic complex.

The perfect man who is a good person a moral character, an exceptional man, a man possessing exceptional or superhuman strength, abilities or powers. Nietzsche's ideal man, according to the philosophy of Nietzsche, an ideal man who through creativity, and integrity is able to transcend good, and evil, and is the goal of human evolution but yet without pity, and showing no mercy, and socialism, a political system of communal ownership of theories, and systems by which the means of productivity, and distribution are controlled by the conscious thought of one aim, and one goal advocating an end to private ownership of property, and exploitation of conscious thought, the stage between capitalism, and communism in the Marxist theory, the stage after the proletarian revolution of the liberation from a moral conscience, and in so they created the reflection of the id the Frankenstein monster, a reflection of their psyche.

And humanism, an idol of worshippers, in the belief in a human based morality, a system of thought, 'If I am I must be,' and so he is, based on the values, theatrics, and behaviors of the beliefs, to be best in human beings, that is the Shakespearian play acted out on the stage of the world, hence the modern Globe theatre of the world for all roads lead to the Holy Roman Empire, rather than on any supernatural authority, hence the sister of the ideological thought of Communism, 'we the people, for we the people,' and so a secular cultural, and intellectual movement of the Renaissance, that spread throughout Europe resulting in two world wars, slavery, the forceful, and bloody colonization of the weaker species on the Global theatre of the Shakespearian existence, Hamlet, Romeo, and Juliet, King Richard, Henry the V, the Tempest, King Lear, in the age old concept of Darwinism, and that survival of the strongest as the main driving force behind Hitler's ideology in exterminating the Jews, like how the Spaniards almost exterminated a civilization in the New World in search of gold, and riches, like how the Americans almost exterminated the American Indian, building the American dream, like how the Australians almost exterminated the native people of that land as a rediscovery of the arts, and philosophy of the thought, 'If I am then I must be,' the ancient Romans, and the ancient Greeks.

And the imperialist believing in the building of an empire based on commerce, the policy of progression of the rule or influence of capitalism over other countries with her political, military, and economic domination of one country over the others, extending its thought, 'If I am then I must be,' to be no more for all roads leads to the Holy Roman Empire, the modern United States of Europe. And shall the one who sees red as black as to the one who sees red as blue the aggressive characteristic of interactions between like minds, usually of the same variety of sequences as we are taught about our past, and so we as students of learning are taught the past of our existence, and in the process our ego, and arrogant natures are revitalized, and so we go out empowered euphorically to try, and save the world when there is nothing really wrong with it accept for those who are trying to change it to save it by blowing it up all the time, making laws that takes away our independence of a free will to serve both God, and man, squandering our natural resources in the pursuit of the American dream, which has now turned into the American nightmare as many begin to see the effect of recession like a serious blood disorder and sometimes fatal like the Vietnam war characterized by a decreased in the coarse show white condition of humanity as it often occurs as a toxic effect of a progression many say from sanity to insanity of the agonistically driven philosopher who is building the molecules of the chemical reaction to give life to this lifeless body of Homo sapiens, the modern story of the Frankenstein monster created by Mary Shelley in her 1818 novel in which the hero creates a living man, a free thinker, free from religions, and all forms of morality to serve king, and country, but instead to serve only me, my wife, and my children, and to hell with the rest of the world Hitlerism who is now the creator of destiny for the modern man, a moral thinking man.

A new species created from the mirror of our perceptions, that there are no absolutes in this modern world, which some of us in authority creates, that causes widespread ruin, and destruction, that he is created to be his own downfall like Hitler, when he took his own life, and became a ghost to many, and to some a martyr, and to some an idealistic God as so you see with the Chinese people as they immortalize his thoughts on paper of Homo sapiens in his book as the modern doctor Frankenstein created an atomically correct creation, that became the maker's downfall as he looses control, and the monster he created becomes, the free thinking modernized man, known as Superman, one of his many of springs, the fascist monster which stopped bombing Britain in 1941 the operation called Sealion, and then out his philosophical complex conscience, like a starving man trying to choose between a well done steak or a leg of roast lamb, in the end he decides that both are desirable, because it is his animalistic nature, that he is trying to gratify, and with both in the mind of a starving man decides, that both are obtainable, and so decides to invades Russia in 1942 in the operation called Barbarossa as his Frankenstein monster created by his own reflection in the mirror of his own horror fairy-tale of what he felt he was, and that was inadequate, as throughout his sad life tried to find out what a real man is as many of us spend all our lives still trying to do, screamed in his morbid conscience for more blood, and widespread destruction came up from the grave where the Frankenstein monster was formed in the imagination of literature, and as a result of this over indulgent imagination, the monster that so stalks us in our darkest hour, that is death without representation or knowing or without warning so that we cannot say goodbye, in an emotional embrace to our love ones as the Grim Reaper, a personification of death approaches.

A cloaked man or skeleton, holding a scythe, now known so commonly as the cape crusader Batman, the saviour of the world, the superhero complex of the id, the theoretical but more so the hidden theatrical hero of our play on the stage called the modern world, as our admirer look on and applauses rain down like summer showers, a part of the human psyche re-discovered by Freud now known as Freudian psychoanalytical theories of the psyche, that is unconscious, and the source of all primitive instinctive impulses, and drives such as murder without conscience, and reason except to gratify our sexual desires, the other part of the psyche, the ego, and the superego, the super hero complex but in the past as the Holy Crusaders who invaded Jerusalem to kill, pillage, and conquer in the name of God, came in as an orgy of violence, and death as so many times before to claimed her prize as she spends based on an agreement with her father Zeus half her time with her husband Hades, and the other half with her mother Demeter, the eternal destiny of Homo sapiens the free thinker, not bound by shame, and guilt of killing a holy man on the cross, the only begotten son of God, or religion, the mind controlling drug of religious zealots who say we must be poor, and suffer under their pious man made laws, that have no life to them, which Christ warned us would come saying, that they are the Christ or any kind of intellectual constraints based on the, 'Law of Moses,' as widely practice in the modern day church as a form of religion of servitude to a written code of practice, that has no life to it and not a relationship with a loving Father who forgives our wrong doing, like a true father does, and sent his only begotten son into the world to show the world how a divine Father relates to his sons, and his daughters, such as with the British government in the Houses of Lord where the men of religion that is the, 'Law of Moses,' argues with the men of philosophy the new conceptual thought of Homo sapiens, in the attempt to create a utopian society of free thinkers, based on economic growth, that is morally correct, in their own eyes, and then returned to oceans of oblivion, the state of forgetfulness of being utterly forgotten unaware of the havoc, and chaos she has created in the destiny to create Homo sapiens, the free thinker of the new world.

The Lake of Fire that burns with Brimstone, Sulphur and Fire. The woman, 'She,' is called Persephone the wife of Hades the Lord of the underworld receives the souls, the ghosts of the dead, that she has slain who are guided by Hermes the messenger God who escorts them to the boatman Charon, who would ferry them across the Styx but only those ghosts who could pay the fare would be allowed to go, those who could indulge her idealism that she is the God of Hades the God of the Lake of Fire, the daughter of Zeus, and Demeter, the earth Goddess as she became the queen of the underworld as the abducted wife of Hades.

Who was promised to him by Zeus himself, and without consulting her mother too. And when Hades took her, Demeter was beside herself with grief as she wondered the earth searching for her daughter, two burning torches in her hands, while the earth was no longer fertile as it is becoming in our present day world, with Global Warming, the opening in the Ozone Layer above us, and the rest who could not pay the fare would roam the earth as vagabond spirits as they communicate with their loved ones through mediums, and psychics as we see on the modern box of our fantasy, to Polydemon the receiver of many guests.

The abode of the rich and famous there they would be met by Cerberus, the three headed dog who guarded the entrance to the underworld known as Hades to make sure no one escapes from the underworld As we mourn our creation of the modern man in our memorials to the slain dead in wars fought for honour. And survival in those famous words that so many mad men's Frankenstein creation since the beginning of time, when man first walked the earth have either thought or said, "only the strong survives." It is the time, and season of the process of natural selection to preserve the pure human race, would just go out into the playing field of the new life of modernism, and create our fantasies on a world stage. Hidden deep within our psyche are these words, 'the world is a stage and I am a play of actors, and actresses, and so I will act out my fantasy, and be adored by the millions of fans who love me as I fulfill my fantasy dream like the fairy tales,' we are taught as children.

Chapter 11

And look at the streams of consciousness the literary style that presents a character's continuous flow of thoughts as they arise from the ashes of the invisible into visible electrical pulses and rhythms that pulsates through one's own veins, like the Phoenix that mythological bird, resembling an eagle that lived for 500 years, and then burned itself to death on a pyre from whose ashes another Phoenix arose the symbol of from death to life to death to life a continuing circle of life, and death, and growth in the past tense, to the future by bypassing this present period of consciousness or progression in the process of evolution of human conscience.

The old age philosopher, and the creation of the intellect, the constellation of the resurrection of the age old eristical argument, the art of disputing against the freedom of the weak, and so the machismo characters of every move of every generation of the development of Homo sapiens, the stereotypical male species on their exaggerated journey of intellect, knowledge, and endless debates that has span the corridors of the development of humanity, emphasizing the characteristics of the typical male hero to try, and save the world by physical strength, courage, aggressiveness, and with the lack of emotional piety.

A religious devotion to our own ego, the strong respectful devotion to the deity of self-belief, and the strict observance of the egotist, the Oedipus complex., a Greek mythological figure a son of Jocasta, and Laius, King of Thebes who unwittingly killed his father, and married his mother. Then being an egotist he puts out his own eyes when he discovered what he had done. Like Hitler, blowing out his brains when he realized what he had done, because of his ego. Later to be known as the Oedipus complex, a theory from the mind of Sigmund Freud, who discovered the unconscious desire for parent's feelings, and desires originating from when a child, more commonly a son unconsciously seeks sexual fulfillment from the parent of the opposite sex. The mechanical rivers of the machine of industrialization, in addition to the jungle concrete ponds, the flora and fauna, the Roman Goddess of flowers, and the ancient Italian Goddess, the sister of Fanus, and the skies considered as a whole process of evolution of the intellectual man. The archaic thought patterns of Homo sapiens reconstituted to form the past in the present a type delusion of sorts. As we see with Oedipus, a son of Jocasta and Laius, later found in the Oedipus complex said to be discovered by Sigmund Freud.

Nevertheless, the conscious of the present whispers into the heart of humanity, the sound of the ages, "it is all the same, nothing ever changes." Look at the words of the righteous preacher, "The thing that hath been, it that which shall be; and that which is done is that which shall be done: and there is no new thing under the sun. For in much wisdom is much grief: and he that increaseth knowledge increaseth sorrow. Then I returned, and I saw vanity under the sun. I said in mine heart concerning the estate of the sons of men, that God might manifest them, and that they might see that they themselves are beasts" The concepts of Darwinism proved true, the story of Homo sapiens the story of evolution. The theory of evolution, first developed by Charles Darwin, the ideology that species of living things originate, evolved, and survive through natural selection in response to the natural elements, that controls the said environment.

We reinvent what has been invented in the past as we travel the corridors of the past to build our future, our past lives of our ancestors who failed at building the Tower of Babel. And so as we get closer to the abomination of desolation, hence the Lucifer ego complex as we hear in the R Kelly Song, I believe I can fly, I believe I can touch the sky, I think about it every night, and day. Going through that open door, just as Lucifer is recording his lyrical song in Isaiah 14: For thou hast said in thine heart, I will ascend into heaven, (I believe I can fly,) I will exalt my throne above the stars of God, (I believe I can touch the sky,) I will sit also upon the mount of the congregation, in the sides of the north; clouds, (I think about it every day,) I will be like the most high, (going through that open door.) As he said, "I will be like the most high," the universe exploded. Hence the heart behind the theory of the scientific theories that the universe began with a great big bang. It was his ego being humbled by the Great Jehovah. His Tower of Babel finally came crashing down on him like the famous nursery rhythm, 'Jack, and Jill went up the hill to fetch a pale of water, and then came tumbling down,' or, 'Humpty Dumpty sat on the wall and suddenly

If I Am Then I Must Be

he fell off and his soldiers could not put him back together again.' In addition, as the devastation comes out of Homo sapiens' hearts when he reaches as far as he is programmed to go.

He explodes as Lucifer did when he became ripe as a stuffed roasted turkey on a roasting stick in a barbecue, like the Lake of Fire his final resting stop. After his thousand years suntan in the bottomless pit stop, hence if God made all life as it is written in the book of Genesis, and saw the future and so he wrote the book of Revelation depicting the end of the world as so many refuse to believe, and so they spend their lives trying to save what has been foretold would be destroyed by the Homo sapiens creation, hence, 'The Hero is Born,' "I will save you," as we have seen throughout the history of the creation of the Homo sapiens from childhood to adulthood. And if God really created all life through Adam and Eve then would he not have designed the Homo sapiens so that he would fail every time he gets close to his goal to create this utopian one world system of Supermen, with no heavenly conscience, like the Holy Roman Empire now called the United States of Europe, which Hitler failed to unite? The Egyptian Empire, The British Empire, and many more that have come and gone defining our future as our past failures relived, and like the wind blows wherever it wills so does the memories of these once so powerful empires goes wherever we will dream. Just as did the explosion that blew up old Lucifer's Tower Of Babel as we find in Ezekiel 28: "Thou hast defiled thy sanctuaries by the multitude of thine iniquities, by the iniquity of thy traffick, therefore will I bring forth a fire from the midst of thee, it shall devour thee, and I will bring thee to ashes upon the earth in the sight of all them that behold thee." The things that I am thinking towards you maybe confusing, but they really are not, it is the blindness of your thoughts, 'If I am then I must be,' that stops you from being who you are for as, 'I become I am,' a little baby born to a mother, and father into a new experience, a different reality experienced than the one I was use to for the nine months in the belly of my mother's womb.

As I listen to the endless sounds of King David's words as they echoed through eternity of the creation in the flesh of Adam's fallen race, "thou compasses my path, and my lying down, and art acquainted with all my ways. For there is not a word in my tongue, but, lo, O Lord Jesus, thou knowest it altogether. Thou hast beset me behind and before, and laid thine hand upon me. Such knowledge is too wonderful for me; it is too high, I cannot attain unto it. 'That I am a son to a divine Father and not a servant to a God like all other Gods of the dust.'"

If I Am Then I Must Be

Chapter 12

That say do as I tell you and not as I do when I showed the whole world how I related in the art of relationship to my son Jesus in the thirty three years that he lived amongst Adam's fallen race, and not a religion, a dead practice of worshipping a written code of practice that no one has ever seen me performed in the written oracles of my relationship with my son Jesus in the earth. Whither shall I go from they Spirit? Or whither shall I flee from thy presence? If I ascend up into heaven, thou art there: if I make my bed in hell, behold, thou art there: if I take the wings of the morning, and dwell in the uttermost parts of the sea; Even there shall thy hand lead, and thy right hand shall hold me. If I say, surely the darkness shall cover me; even the night shall be light about me.

Yea, the darkness hides about me. Yea, the darkness hides not from thee; but the light shines as the day: the darkness, and the light are both alike to thee. For thou hast possessed my reins: thou hast covered me in my mother's womb. I will praise thee; for I am fearfully and wonderfully made: 'as science is beginning to discover,' marvelous are thy works; and that my soul knoweth right well. My unformed substance was not hid from thee, when I was made in secret, and curiously wrought in the lowest parts of the earth. Thine eyes did see my unformed substance, yet being imperfect; and in thy book of life all my members were written, which in continuance were fashioned, when as yet there was none of them. How precious also are thy thoughts unto me, O God Jesus! And this is your thought to me: For the preaching of the cross is to them that perish, foolishness; but unto us, which are saved it, is the power of the Jehovah God the Great I AM That I AM, for it is written. I will destroy the wisdom of the wise, and will bring to nothing the understanding of the prudent. And so I say to you wise men of the earth you men of intellect, you men of philosophy, you men of learning, you men of science, you men of religion, where is the great Egyptian Empire? Where is the great Babylon Empire? Where is the great Holy Roman Empire? Where is the great British Empire? Where is the wise? Where is the scribe? Where is the disputer of this world? For after that is the wisdom of God Jehovah the world by wisdom knew not God the great Jehovah the life force of that which is alive and of all that is dead in the sea of forgetfulness hath not Jehovah made foolish the wisdom of this world? That man is a moral thought."

The Third Reich, the Aryan nation or more bluntly as we see it in the heroic complex, the perfect man who is a good person a moral character, an exceptional man, a man possessing exceptional or superhuman strength, abilities or powers. Nietzsche's ideal man, according to the philosophy of Nietzsche, an ideal man who through creativity and integrity is able to transcend good and evil, and is the goal of human evolution, but yet without pity and showing no mercy, for after that in the wisdom of Jehovah the world by true wisdom knew not the great Jehovah instead creating the scientist to explain in the wisdom of Adam's fallen race, what is already known to man so it pleased the great Jehovah by the foolishness of preaching of the cross to save them that believe. For the Jews require a sign, and the Greeks seek after wisdom: But we preach Christ crucified, unto the Jews an obstacle, and the Greeks foolishness; But unto them, which are called, both Jews, and Greeks, Christ the power of the great Jehovah, and his wisdom.

Because the foolishness of Jehovah is wiser than men, such as spending millions of dollars to put a dead piece of metal into space to search for life when the life of those who their ancestors robbed to build their economic revolution, such as the slave trade as they traveled the Atlantic Salve route, are dying from the lack of food, and the sounds of the modern man the moral Homo sapiens is silent as their conscience grows dead to the sounds of the ages whispers, 'Where is your compassion for the dying? Where is your mercy in the wars that you fight killing those who do not see like you?' Thus creating the modern Homo sapiens, who creates peace by shedding the blood of all those who will not conform to the image of the Beast, the commerce of the modern world, and the weakness of the great Jehovah is stronger than men. For ye see your calling, brethren, how that not many wise men after the flesh, not many mighty, not many noble, are called. Both the great Jehovah hath chosen the weak things of the world to confound the things, which are mighty." The Third Reich, the Aryan nation or more bluntly, as we see it in the heroic complex, the perfect man who is a good person a moral character, an exceptional man, a man possessing

If I Am Then I Must Be

exceptional or superhuman strength, abilities or powers. Nietzsche's ideal man, according to the philosophy of Nietzsche, an ideal man who through creativity and integrity is able to transcend good and evil and is the goal of human evolution, but yet without pity, and showing no mercy, Saturn's religious men's, last attempt to stop the work of human compassion going any further, and that is not the work of separatism or division as the western church portrays a relationship with the Father, but the gospel of reconciliation for all humanity no matter what background you are from, but it has failed.

As I stopped ruminating for a while I begin to think on what I am coming to, and that is to a point where I do not care much about worldly things anymore as much as I do care more about heavenly things as portrayed in all life, including humanity, animals, nature, and life in general. I have been doing some soul searching, and I have seen where I have made the mistakes, that have caused my passions not to honour my promises in my life. Now I am about to correct them. And as King David finished his reflection upon the greatness of his, and my God he says, "And the based things of the world, and things which are despised, hath Jehovah chosen yea, and things which are not to bring to naught things that are. That no flesh should glory in his presence. But of him are ye in Christ Jesus, who of the great Jehovah is made unto us wisdom, and righteousness, and sanctification, and redemption. How great is the sum of them! If I should count them, they are more in number than the sand: when I awake, I am still with thee." And I am as I am born into a world of sight, sound, thought, speech, touch, smell, and taste, and taught to forget who I was before I came into awareness of who I really am, to be who I am to be for, 'If I am then I must be.' And so my brainwashing begins, for as I enter the training camps of logic I am brainwashed into believing in the past failures of the modern Homo sapiens. I am retrained in the school of thought to accept the intellectual ideas of fallen men, the Homo sapiens who are trapped in the prison of time. Thus, the term called, 'Ground Hog Day.' His frustration at his own mortality and frailty, his weakness, his susceptibility to catch diseases, and waste away in fear of the unknown, hence twelve hours to perceive the light of day, twelve hours to go the neither land, which is neither here or there just a dream as I dream of what I want to be, to be told suddenly that I am a number a national insurance number, a identity card, a passport, a commodity in the statistics of government policy, and not a individual human being, finally becoming as I stood upon the sand of the seas, and saw a Beast rise up out of the sea having seven heads, and ten horns, and upon his horns ten crowns, and upon his heads the name of blasphemy. And the Beast, which I saw, was like unto a leopard, and his feet were as the feet of a bear, and his mouth as the mouth of a lion, and the dragon gave him power, and his seat, and great authority. And I saw one of his heads as it were wounded to death; and his deadly wound was healed: and all the world wondered after the Beast. And they worshipped the worship the concept of ego the creation of the alto ego the Frankenstein monster brought to life in the literary forms of creation as Uther Pendragon forms in the imagination of the literary writer the process of natural selection, only the most strongest, and savage Homo sapiens survives in the process of evolution as he battles against the Duke of Cornwall as Merlin fulfils his promise to beguile to him as he wins, and holds his attention, the Frankenstein monster of the past, the ancient dragon taking human form, in his interest, and devotion to be mislead, and deceived, and robbed of the literary ending of all that all hero seek, and that is of the, 'Sword of Power,' 'Excalibur,' to unite the ethos of the Holy Roman Empire, a man without conscience, pity, compassion, and mercy to the indifferent of all other species of life.

A man without supernatural intelligence like the Third Reich, the Aryan nation or more bluntly, as we see it in the heroic complex, the perfect man who is a good person a moral character, an exceptional man, a man possessing exceptional or superhuman strength, abilities or powers. Nietzsche's ideal man, according to the philosophy of Nietzsche, an ideal man who through creativity and integrity is able to transcend good, and evil, and is the goal of human evolution but yet without pity, and showing no mercy, Saturn's religious men's, last attempt to denote the kingship of all Empires, and so Merlin retrieves the sword from the, 'Lady of the Lake.' who is the alto ego of Jezebel the Mystery Harlot, and beguiles it to Uther Pendragon with the deceptive intentions of misleading the Dragon in human form in the intention of uniting the land as one for all roads leads to Rome, 'the Holy Roman Empire,' the confederate states of the renovated, 'United Europe,' Rome reborn. After the Dragon in human form yields portions of that which was given to all humanity without the consent of all those who lived, and lives on it and make their living from it as the land produces true life, hence a cow, which only feeds on grass, and water but yet to the natural man the cow gives milk, cheese, butter, curd, cream, beef, steak, and much more for free, and so the children of the Dragon those who have taken, 'The Mark of The Beast,' the mark of commerce, takes the freedom of the land, and so make commerce in their industrial revolution to produce a system of credit, and turn the inhabitants of the free land into economic slaves to the Beast of commerce as they sell out their integrity of being what is human for commerce, and that as the Politicians would say creates jobs that leads nowhere as the slaves of the Beast work themselves into the grave with long hours of sheer boredom never really seeing the glorious land of hope, and in the tradition of the Dragon taking what is not rightfully his, and then giving it as a bargaining tools to whoever he pleases to as they make secret treaties for all the nations have drunk of the blood wine of the wrath of her fornication, and the kings of the earth have committed fornication with her, and the merchants of commerce of the earth are waxed rich through the abundance of her delicacies. And I heard another voice from heaven, saying, and he cried from heaven having great power, and the earth was lightened with his glory, come out of her, my people that ye be not partakers of her sins, and that ye receive not of her plagues. For her sins have reached unto heaven, and the great judge of all humanity hath remembered her iniquities. And now has rewarded her even as she has rewarded you, and double unto her double according to her works: in the cup with, which she hath filled, Pandora's Box, fill to her double.

How much she hath glorified herself, and lived deliciously, so much torment, and sorrow she has caused in the earth therefore shall her plagues come in one day, death, and mourning, and famine; and she shall be utterly burned with fire: for strong is the Lord God Jehovah who judgeth her. And the kings of the earth, who have committed fornication, and lived deliciously with her, shall bewail her, and lament for her, when they shall see the smoke of her burning. Standing afar off or the fear of her torment, saying, Alas, alas that great city Babylon, Rome, Troy, Camelot, Egypt, Assyria, the Tower of London, the Kremlin, that mighty city! For in one hour is thy judgment come. And the merchants of the earth shall weep and mourn over her; for no man buyeth their merchandise anymore. The merchandise of gold, and silver, and precious stones, and of pearls, and fine linen, and purple and silk, and scarlet, and all thine wood, and all manner vessels of most precious wood, and of brass, and iron, and marble, and cinnamon, and odours, and ointments, and frankincense, and wine, and oil, and fine flour, and wheat, and beasts, and sheep, and horses and chariots, and slaves, and souls of men. And the fruits that thy soul lusted after are departed from thee, and all things, which were dainty, and goodly, are departed from thee, and thou shalt find them no more at all.

The merchants of these things, which were made rich by her, shall stand afar off for the fear of her torment, weeping and wailing, and saying, as one famous modern merchant once said, I did not know we were in a recession, alas, alas that great city, that was clothed in fine linen, and purple, and scarlet, and decked with gold, and precious stones, and pearls. For in one hour so great riches is come to naught like the billions that have come to naught in the banks' mad pursuit of her luxuries. And every shipmaster and all the company in ships, and sailors, and as many as trade by sea, stood afar off, and cried when they saw the smoke of her burning, saying, what city is like unto this great city! 'Kingdoms from here to the sea of all nations,' Cornwall yields to the Dragon in human form as he promises to enforce the great Beast's will. And the beguiled, and enchanted Cornwall invites the Beast to dine in the celebration of that old secret treaty, the destiny of men's souls within his fortress of solitude where the race of Supermen goes, and as the Beast sees, and becomes wild with the lustful passion of his real nature, the nature of a Beast untrained in the etiquette of the modern hero as he is enchanted by Cornwall's wife Igrayne. And so Cornwall yields to his animalistic nature for we all evolved from a lesser form of the Homo sapiens, are angered, and so the pack with Beasts, and men is at an end.

The Dragon now lays siege to his lustful passions of the moral man. 'If I am then I must be,' and so encircles the Duke' castle. And then the cunningly Merlin, agrees to use his magic tricks of illusions, and delusions to seduce Igrayne, beguiling him, and so misleading the Dragon in human form to his death, robbing him of the hero's fairy tale ending. So Merlin summons another but greater dragon, which lies beneath the land and transforms Uther the slain Dragon into the reflection of the light of his own perception, the image of Cornwall, who rides into the castle across the sky on the dragon's breath just as Cornwall leaves to attack Uther's camp. The dragon, which gave power unto the Beast: and they worshipped the Beast, saying, who is like unto the Beast? Who is able to make war with him? And there was given unto him a mouth speaking great things, and blasphemies; and power was given unto him to continue forty, and two months. And he opened his mouth in blasphemy against the Lord of the heavens to blaspheme his name, and his tabernacle, and them that dwell in heaven. And it was given unto him to make war with the saints, and to overcome them: and power was given him over all kindred, tongues, and nations. And all that dwell upon the earth shall worship him, whose names are not written in the, 'book of life of the Lamb,' slain from the foundation of the world. If any man have an ear let him hear. He that is led into captivity shall go into captivity; he that kills with the sword must be killed with the sword. Here is the patience, and the faith of the saints. And I beheld another Beast coming up out of the earth, and he had two horns like a lamb, and he spake as a dragon. And he exercise all the power of the first Beast before him, and causes the earth, and them which dwell therein to worship the first Beast whose deadly wound was healed, and he doeth great wonders, so that he makes fire come down from heaven like Elijah of ancients times, in the sight of men and deceives them that dwell on the earth by the means of those miracles, which he had power to do in the sight of the Beast; saying to them that dwell on the earth, that they should make an image to the Beast, it is called commerce, and industrial growth, which had the wounds of recession by the sword and did live.

And he had power to give life unto the image of commerce as he injected the tax payer's capital into the failing banking systems of the world's economies, the Beast, that the image of the Beast should both speak, and cause that as many as would not worship the image of the Beast should be killed. The homeless, the poor starving victims of war, famine, and poverty, those who had not taken, 'The Mark of The Beast,' that is commerce without a conscience, the greed, and lust of the world, those who make commerce by exploiting the vulnerable, calling it freedom of speech but without the moral responsibility of those famous words of liberty, long forgotten by economic growth that goes something like, "I am free to do whatever I want without the maturity, and the adult responsibility of not influencing the less liberated than I to kill, murder, or to cause harm to the delicate, and fragile minds of the vulnerable, that are so easily influenced by their peers into doing wrong, thus ruining their lives for a pound, a dollar, in the famous line I buy that for a dollar," and they have no representation in governments, because they do not create wealth, honour, and national pride, to give encouragement to the fool, that believes the Homo sapiens is the ultimate modern creation from the imagination of fallen man. So that governments, that governs their affairs could boast in the arena of boastings, that our people are the great people of the world the Aryan philosophy that created the race of Superheroes in the first place, with an amoral conscience but without mercy, pity and empathy for the weak and the undesirables as they say to these oppressive regimes the forms of governmental styles especially those considered to be brutal, and oppressive adopting a management style of the Victorian Empire, "If they won't obey us then kill them, and enslave them for we are the law, because we kill with metal bullets, and cannons those who kill with sticks and string in their bow, and arrows." Hence the father of Charles Darwin's theory of natural selection, the survival of the fittest, hence, 'who dares wins.'

That first you must have a political system that allows for each member of your country to vote, and they must be able to choose their leaders, which is their democratic right as the moral thinker thinks; the humanist in his moral consciousness, the perfect man who is a good person a moral character, an exceptional man, a man possessing exceptional or superhuman strength, abilities or powers. Nietzsche's ideal man, according to the philosophy of Nietzsche, an ideal man who through creativity the Renaissance era, and integrity is able to transcend good and evil, and is the goal of human evolution, but yet without pity, and showing no mercy, while those who these modern day humanistic humanitarians are to get the democratic right to vote in choosing their own governments are dying from diseases such as cholera, and starvation, while the democratic governments, the pride of the modern Homo sapiens is arguing in the ethos of the age old argument of the management style of the Victorian Empire, "if they won't obey then kill them and

If I Am Then I Must Be

enslave them for we are the law of a moral, and ethical people, that will let the innocent, and weak, the third world people die of starvation so that we can look good as a democratic nation, thus promoting a more better government, that allows everyone the right to vote," and so in modern governments morality is judged by how well you pass your math and English exams so that Politicians can boast, that the race of Homo sapiens; the Third Reich reborn, the Aryan race, now the progressing evolving nations evolving into the modern world, the new prison of time and space, the seed of Cain, that wicked one who murdered his own brother out of jealousy, and pride the id-sub conscious monster now brought to life by Mary Shelly, in the her alto ego Frankenstein, like the mild mannered alto ego of Karl El known as Clark Kent, the Superman syndrome or more bluntly as we see it in the heroic complex in our mind's eye the visual imagination and memory the place where visual images are conjured up like magic tricks to frill the audiences, conjured up from the memory of renovations of the reconstitution of why I exist, like a renovation of a dilapidated old building of thought, taste, touch, sight and sound.

In the container of interpretations of a different kind but the same building of the imagined scene a mental constructed picture of thought, taste, touch, sight and sound. As the artist of rendition recreates what has been, and has already been done in the past in a mental scene constructed from the memory of the imagination on the theatrical stage called the world, where thought, taste, touch, sight, and sound becomes visible from the invisible realm of the unconscious soul. And so comes forth on the stage of life the perfect man who is a good person a moral character, an exceptional man, a man possessing exceptional or superhuman strength, abilities or powers. Nietzsche's ideal man, according to the philosophy of Nietzsche, an ideal man who through creativity, the arts and integrity is able to transcend good, and evil, and is the goal of human evolution but yet without pity, and showing no mercy, Saturn's religious men's, last attempt to stop the work of true human compassion as he said as Pilate said unto him, "Art thou a king then?" and human compassion answered. "Thou sayest that I am a king. To this end I was born, and for this witness unto the truth. Every one that is of the truth heareth my voice." Pilate saith unto the true human compassion, "what is truth?" And then as time goes by and decades comes and goes, like the wind that is neither here or there but everywhere for just a moment, even in centuries of war and violence, famines and plagues, and diseases Jack Nicholson on the world's stage the Globe theatre of acting out our literary perceptions, of what we are thinking about ourselves, finally answers Pilate's age old question, that has plaque the conscience of the Homo sapiens for six thousand years of conscious thought as the moral man breathes, and denotes in his dead conscience his words, as he remembers them when he spoke them two thousand years ago revealing his true nature, and the point of unbearable pressure as he screamed at Pilate, and he answered, and says, "human compassion's blood be on us, and our children," Jack Nicholson answers Pilate's question in the famous Hollywood theatrical performance a play called, 'A Few Good Men,' and he answers back through the corridors of time echoed from upon the stage of the world in the theatre of the universal dream, 'If I am then I must be,' 'and to be no more.' As he screams at Tom Cruise, "You can't handle the truth." And when he had said this, he went out again unto the political systems of the world still in the loins of the Jews and the Gentiles for a nation starts as two people, one male, and one female as they procreate in the joyful union of sex to procreate a race of nations, like Adam and Eve the parents of modern man, hence the fallen man, the DNA of man, the modern man the Homo sapiens. And as scientists learn more about what is, and will always be in the mutations in the DNA of people, that exist in the entire world, geneticists are finding out more about the humans who have populated the Earth.

These facts leads to the modern day African, and so it is now known that the DNA of the modern day African is more diverse than of all the people from other nations establishing, that the statement, demonstrating, that humans have lived there the longest is in fact true. And now proves the hypothesis, that the ancient African genes is found in all human races existing today, and so Pilate saith unto them Saying, "that I find no fault at all. But yet ye have a custom that I should release unto you one at the Passover: will ye therefore that I release unto you the King of the human compassion the Jew?" "Not this man they replied, but the murderer, and thief Barabbas." Then answered all the people, and said, "His blood be on us, and our children." Then Pilate released he that is Barabbas unto them: and when he had scourged human compassion, such as he scourged Martin Luther King Jr, Abraham Lincoln, Gandhi, and even Jesus Christ, he delivered them to be crucified. And the truth that humanity cannot handle is that they cannot change, and that it takes to be born from above to change, and so anyone who comes into the human world's prison, to show them what we really are, and that are animals, they kill, and then they make commerce from his or her death by developing experts on how these liberators lived. The greatest of them all was Christ but he came back from the dead to everyone surprise. Then going any further, came the work of separatism or division as the western church portrays a relationship without the Father, the gospel of reconciliation for all humanity, no matter what background they are from but it has failed, because, 'If I am then I must be,' is coming to a point where I do not care anymore, and so I will pursue worldly things. As the literary artist changes his literary work to, 'I care little about heavenly things as portrayed in all my life's work,' including humanity, animals, nature, and life in general. "I have been doing some soul searching, and I have seen where I have made the mistakes, that I have caused. Now I am about to correct them." Therefore, he causes all, both small and great, rich and poor, free and bond to receive a mark in their right hand, or in their foreheads.

In addition, that no man might buy or sell, save he that had the mark, or the name of the Beast, or the number of his name. an id card, a passport, a national insurance number, a criminal record, insurance details, a bank card, a credit card, a credit agreement, a credit history, a driver's license, a loan statement, a crime report, an email address, a phone number, here is wisdom. Let him that hath understanding count the number of the Beast: for it is the number of a man; and his number is six hundred threescore, and six, 'The Mark of The Beast,' 666, hence wealth, wealth, wealth, three lots of six letter syllables, that equal the number 18 the name of the Antichrist. Hence the ideology of I have found out who has a right to live, and not just survive as a national insurance number, or a id card, or a passport, a criminal record, insurance details, a bank card, a credit card, a credit agreement, a credit history, a driver's license, a loan statement, a crime report, an email address, a phone number but as a citizen of creationism, and then again eleven years to be a child, then another eleven years of teenage hood, then about twenty years of being a young man, then another twenty years of being a middle aged man, then maybe if I am lucky, about another twenty years as a old man then my time has run out as I look into the hour glass of my reality for as the heaven is high above the earth, so great is his mercy toward them that fear him. As far as the east is from the west, so far hath he removed our transgressions from us. Like a father pities his children, so human mercy, the Lord pities them that fear him. For he knows our frame; he remembers that we are dust. As for man, his days are as grass: as a flower of the field, so he flourishes. For the wind of change blows steadily over him, and he is gone, and the place thereof shall no him no more, all goes dark a sad end to my journey of awareness of sight a world of sight, sound, thought, speech, touch, smell and taste, taught to forget who I was before I came into awareness of who I really am, to be who I am to be for, 'If I am then I must be.' As I draw my last breath at the applauses as the curtains come down and the performance ends in the Globe theatre of the world. With raving reviews from critics, and as one famous very famous performer said to his critics, "History will be the judge of whether it was a good decision to go to war." For it to start all over again, another child is born to take my place in the great experiment of the perfect Frankenstein monster the humanist, and their idol, the new, and improved Homo sapiens, the modern day Clark Kent with his alto ego Karl El so commonly seen on the battlefields of wars throughout generation thru generation.

The Third Reich, the Aryan nation, the Holy Roman Empire, queen Victoria's England, the ideologies of the Pope, or more bluntly as we see it in the heroic complex. The perfect Homo sapiens man who is an accomplished expert of moral character, an extraordinary man, a man possessing special or Herculean strength, abilities or powers. Nietzsche's ideal man, according to the philosophy of Nietzsche, an ideal man who through inspiration and honour is able to transcend good, and evil, and is the goal of human evolution but yet without pity, and showing no mercy, Saturn's sacred men's, last attempt to stop the work of creationism going any further, and that is not the work of separatism or division as the western church portrays a relationship without the Father, and the gospel of reconciliation for all humanity no matter what background they are from.

Chapter 13

Awakes the childless creation of the union of Igrayne and his wife, Morgana the eunuch paralyzed by the castration of her mother's virtue by the Homo Erectus the male sex organ of a man's body who can only think with his testicles like my father, Uther' the dragon in human form as the Beast. Or more rather, 'the Homo,' a word that comes from the Latin language, 'Homo,' meaning man as pertaining to the species under the genre of, 'Homo,' and includes the in existence, and wiped out species of humans, long gone, like the rejects, that we throw away, after we have finished with them, breathes upon Morgana's mother in his disguised as Igrayne, which is a skill, that I have heard, that witches, and Politicians possess, and so later gives birth, a young daughter, in male form, for men are the embodiments of ego the Homo Erectus, in Dragon form, the Beast reborn as he reinvents himself, in our dreams, desires, hopes as we watch in the theatre of life, hence the Global theatre, life the perception of our reflection of the modern man, 'If I am then I must be,' and so comes forth the new, and improved model, like the brand new Ford automobile as it rolls of the production line, into service, only to be discarded, when the owner is either bored of the use of this once brand new automobile or because it has passed it sell by date.

The modern version of the Homo sapiens, while women as the embodiment of wisdom, that is an empty hollow sound of endless regret, and cries of woes as they see the Politicians play the opinion of yourself game, with their children's lives, after the day of giving birth to a sparkling soul in the image of a cute little baby, then spending all their working lives, looking after that child, teaching him right, and wrong, feeding him, sending him to primary school, then to secondary school, then to college, then even maybe to university, and then the Politicians sending them of to fight for their sense of self, on the battlefield, believing in some speech, that the Politicians gives about national pride, and that we are men, and so being men, we must sacrifice our lives, for a thought of indifference to another thought of indifference, and so by murdering, we can bring peace, and if this was the right way forward, then wars would not keep happening, one after the other, one after the other, one after other, and so it goes on, without end, an endless, and endless journey, into self-image, which is a reflection of self-worth, just like the second generation of Titians overthrew their parents, and imprisoned them, for their self-worth. Therefore, it is with their children as we try to emulate the God's of Mount Olympus. In our fantasies, in our dreams, in our nightmares, and in our aspirations of what we call governing our self-interest.

As the Superhero Politicians tries to save the world, with their policies of endless hope, and the funny thing is, with all the education, they have all the degrees, all the PhDs, yet they cannot see one simple problems, if their policy have not brought about the great, and allusive utopia, that so many Politicians both past, and present have dreamed of, and tried to build, and Politicians have existed for thousands of years, then is it logical to continue on the same path? When it has never been proven, that it actually works? Kind of like the old age debate on whether the devil, and his demons will ever win a battle against the human condition of the soulical realm of existence, and they have been debating this for longer than man has existed, trying to build this great utopian society of logical thought, and that is, 'if I am a good person then I must be a moral person,' the concept of, 'If I am then I must be,' and so I am only to be gone from being to existing after about I would say seventy years, to the land of, 'I was to be no more,' the land of Polydemon, the underworld For, 'If I am then I must be,' then I am, and so I have created in my own image of, 'I am then I must be.' One sense of the word my destiny and that is the grave, where the fruits and rewards of my perception of the colour red, the disturbing opaque colour black, where there is no light of day. No stars, no clouds, just opaque black, the end of being.

In addition, the emotionless blue. The natural colours of the rainbow, forever a fading memory of the natural colours of the creationistic mysticism, the writing of fiction, poetry, or even drama are exercised as all are put into a position of being unable to understand or explain the mysteriously opaque black darkness, that is so hard to understand, for there is nothing to see, nothing to perceive anymore, for the light of the reflection of Homo sapiens is now extinguished by the sudden coming of the opaque black, the

If I Am Then I Must Be

darkness, and so perception cannot be perceived in Polydemon, which awaits me, and where the wealthy make their abode. What good is money, riches and fame in the darkness, where no light is seen, and is never to be to seen or heard of again? Where reflection is no more, so perception dies, and becomes an empty vast ocean of emotions in the deep blue sea of endless regret as the illusion of perception is finally realized. In addition, this is why, why did I exist? The word what did I live for in the light of perception. As the rich ruler tormented by the opaque black, the darkness of his once dead soul, now rotting a rotting diseased corpse stands alone in the darkness as no light can be shed on his quandary as he looks on the light bearer Abraham, the father of the Jews and the Gentile nations, those who saw in the light of truth. And obeyed as he said "I am the way, the truth, and the life, no one come to the Father but through me, and if you believe in me you shall walk in the light, and never again walk in the darkness of the reflection of perception in the mirror of belief in intuitive soulish revelation, the belief that personal communication or union, with the vague opaque black of the darkness of our souls, and lustful desires is the way to enlightenment, and liberation from, 'the Law of Creation,' " as so many have tried to change, through the mirror of perception, by perceiving, that they are, and therefore must be, like the murderer who is sentenced to death, screaming in his heart, unseen from the eyes of curiosity, "I do not want to die," but yet is powerless to stop his execution, for it is the Law, and the Law must be obeyed, by everyone.

As the rich ruler's corrupted, conscience begs for frivolousness light, in the darkness, so that his perception, in the mirror of understanding of self can once again be seen. As the famous wise man, the son of God, and the son of man said, "What does it profit a man to gain the whole world, and loose his soul in the darkness of self, the land of Polydemon, where the emptiness, and endless regret, and the gnashing of teethes resides. What does it profit's the rich to enter the hot overwhelming oceans of Polydemon, never to return to the land of the living, the land of light for Cerberus, the three headed dog, who guards the entrance to the underworld known as Hades, will not let them leave this place of opaque black, and blue emotions, where they are escorted by the boatman Charon, who would ferry them across the Styx but only those ghosts who could pay the fare, would be allowed to go," and the fare is this as a young wise man once wrote in, "and this is the condemnation, that light is come into the world, and men loved darkness rather than light, because their deeds were evil. For every one that doeth evil hates the light neither comes to the light, lest his deeds should be reproved."

And so those who could indulged in their reflection of lust, and decadence, their idealism that she is the chosen path answered, found in and then answered all the people, and said, "his blood be on us, and our children." And so Charon does as he did, When Pilate saw, that he could prevail nothing, but rather tumult was made, he took water, and washed his hands, before the multitude, saying, "I am innocent of the blood of this just man: see ye to it."

If I Am Then I Must Be

Chapter 14

As soon as nobody, with half of the end of good judgment, of the central anxious system, calculated by brainwave, through the leisure interest on an electroencephalogram, over a set period of time, since its occurrence, can allow the termination of the life support or the removal of organs for transmission to a new plantation of Homo sapiens as the modern man tries to go beyond an offensive term, meaning of extremely low intellectual abilities, the anatomy of the appendage of thoughts of feelings, the controlling centre of the panicky system in versatility of the connection to the Darwinism, the tree of life, the spinal cord of the anatomy of the discord of harmony in the enclosed head of the philosopher's moral effects, consisting of a mass of nerve tissue, and nerve supporting, and de-nourishing tissues, the centre of thoughts, and emotions, and regulates bodily activities, and unable to stop thinking about the questions, that so allude the modern man, and so the brain of intellectual pursuit of the word, 'being,' becomes a beating heart in the violently turmoil of the intellect, nourishing the agonistic nature of the Homo sapiens, trying to affect evolution, in an effect of appearing manufactured like the manufactured automobile as it is assembled on the assembly line of progression, into a better society of thought, 'If I am then I must be,' an exaggerated literary argumentative of the Renascences of Europe, that tends to argue, and is eager to win the argument of the tree of life, that just cannot exist in the absolute reality, made up of non realities, instead of the reflections of the perceptions, that we see in the mirrors of life.

And the human condition, the Lord God commanded conscious thought contained in the earth of creation, a part of a whole part, in one part, hence a conscious fraction contained in time, for it was spoken, that time shall only be one hundred twenty years, for thought, and that is to be, that which I think am, and then it will be no more but a fading memory, like the fading sunset as it fades into the winter night of stars, and bright clouds of the night's cosmos far, far away, like a dream, that when we wake up from in the bright morning of the light of our perception of our own reflection, in the mirror of life, it is gone without a goodbye, my sweet lullaby, in the minds of the young who are trying to save the world, in the saying of the Nietzsche Superman, of every tree of the garden, "thou may freely eat, but of the tree of the knowledge of good and evil, the thought, 'If I am then I must be,' thou shall not eat of it, for in the day, that thou eats thereof thou shall surely be, that which, that is, and no more shall thou be, and the fruits there of, you shall be," and so conscious thought, contained in the container of the earth of creation did, and from his loins came Homo sapiens, 'If I am then I must be,' to be no more, just a fading memory of the imagination of the race of Supermen of intellectual thoughts, and ideals through poetry, literature, theatre and of course not forgetting Shakespeare, trying to bring peace to the world, by creating wars, famines, starvation, disease, poverty, illness, servitude, slavery, decadence, crime, by the policies, that they make but in truth all conscious thought, contained in the containers of dust, for all think alike, a car is a car to the Chinese, the Indians, the Hispanics, the Americans, the Europeans, the Jews, the Arab and the American Indians, and in so all relative conceptual thoughts of every single nation on this earth, have the same names for the same experience, that every single person on this earth encounters, in their existence of touch, taste, see, smell, and hear, consumed, from the tree of knowledge of good, and evil.

From their loins came Nazism, Imperialism, Communism, Democracy, Humanism, Feminism, Marxism, Sarcasm, Homosexuality, Bestiality, and much more, and so if they cannot pull of the big revolution, and create a new kind of utopia, then why do Politicians think they can? So the older masculine Homo sapiens, often act out their fantasies as Titians, contradictory to the great majority of their younger version, only in the sums materiality, because the giant Titians can only reproduce, what they are, and so in old age, and in their experience of cynical changes, their physical condition is regarded as comparatively motionless, and so the medical recorders are learning through the boy to man experience, stands on the plane of an assortment of hereditarily development, and as they become, what they are, by being what they are not, in a sense, an understanding of thoughts, becomes what they are not, it is called intellect, and factors out the expression of creativity of an inner world, that looks at the outside world, in the eyes of an infant, thus making new discoveries, in their imaginations everyday, and so in the process of thought – learning, hence the ethos of bringing out the treasures buried within the heart of this student, who is learning to see through the eyes of an infant, new conceptions, for the modern man to explore, instead of just repeating the past, in the hope that the Titian's sense of self, will be smoothed.

When a meticulously single sperm struggles in one moment of a defining moment, slides its way addictively into an anticipation of a sexually charge atoms, thus procreating a life form, a baby is beginning, developing into Mary Shelly's alto ego of her Frankenstein monster, hence everything, that she hated about herself, projected in her relationship with men, made flesh, in literary form, hence probably the founding Titian, in the motherly form of the Feminist movement, is projected into a mass of Y chromosome, determining the male sex of a Homo Erectus, the primitive form of the Homo sapiens, the modern man

The horizontally, vertical axis, in three dimensional form standing vertically with different curves, and shapes, and colours, the defining moment of a joining of two hearts beating as one, in the union of an intimately sexual expression, that produces sperms to carry on the thought of the Titians as they procreate their species of the Super race of future Titians, who will one day rule the world, hence the moral man, the modern Homo sapiens. The male blueprint for the often misfortunate beginning of the muscular genetically altered architecturally man, by logical thought from boy as a baby boy is born into a world, free of any analytical expressions, that age old ability of logic, that is 'true by meaning alone,' without looking where it came from, where it is leading all humanity, what is its shortfalls, and has it ever worked, thus bringing about real change inside the conscience of humanity, slowly regresses into the male adult blueprint, thus beginning to be suppressed in their emotions, that leads to emotional problems later in life, suggesting, that the masculine male archetype, the originally sound model of the ancient man, the Homo Erectus Male is just, the same model as the modern man, hence the Homo sapiens but just differently engineered as to seem brand new, like in modern academic writing style, that is found in writing an essay, 'the song is an archetype of the original composition of classical music, created in the mid 18th century.' Then onto nursery school, then onto primary school, then onto secondary school, then onto university, then onto a brand new career, that turns into the same boring old job, then onto retirement, then onto the grave, then onto to his final resting place Polydemon, the underworld. It is called the progression of the modern day society, where everyone is an individual national insurance number, of a lot of national insurance numbers, and so when one of the national insurance numbers goes to the Social Security Office, he is referred to as a national insurance number, and not an infant, who has grown into adulthood as King David once said, "for thou possessed my reins: thou hast covered me in my mother's womb.

I will praise thee; for I am fearfully and wonderfully made: marvellous are thy works; and that my soul knows right well. My substance was not hid from thee, when I was made in secret, and curiously wrought in the lowest parts of the earth. Thine eyes did see my substance, yet being unperfect; and in thy book all my members were written, which in continuance were fashioned, when as yet there was none of them. How precious also are thy thoughts unto me, O man of true compassion! How great is the sum of them! If I should count them, they are more in number than the sand; when I awake from sleep, I am still with thee," but as the direly, and very badly written of, as she begins, serve as a seriously, and desperately looking customer service reprehensive assistant, for the government of the Antichrist' department, looks him squarely in the eyes, and repeats what she has been trained to do, in the school of logical thought, " here is wisdom let him that hath understanding count the number of a national insurance number, it is the number of a man; and his number is Six hundred threescore and six. And if you do not have this national insurance number that is a number of a man, you will not be able to buy or sell, save unless, that you have this national insurance number, 'the Mark of the Beast,' of commerce, and economic development of the golden age of industrialization for this is the name of progression to a better society, hence the name of the Beast now called Capitalism, Imperialism, Communism, and so on." And on the playground of life, and learning, boys tend to resist singing in performance, in front of the girls, thus controlling the language, and facilitates of the socialization of both sexes as they intermingle with each other so perhaps underdeveloped. In school and so excelling at the mathematics of modern day life and that is the boys have a tendency to excel at the task of hiding their vulnerability, and other tasks controlled by the right side of the brain. The natural aptitudes of the mucho erotic hero, the prodigy of the family of Titians, strengthened by the testosterone of the male narcissistic nature of the psycho's psyche, the Homo Erectus, thus making up the rules as they ago along, trying to become, 'the Modern day Homo sapiens,' the testaments of modern life, affects the boys, and becomes their development, for the most part noticeable during puberty, a harsh call, of brute force, begins to forms the baby flesh, and the male testosterones are mostly responsible for the harmonious development of the chaos as they behave like wild animals, fighting in the streets instead of dancing in the streets as a joyous celebration of different life styles, and cultures but instead in anger, and racism, they kill each other as a sign of respect, and what is there to respect in death?

But the pain of the lost ones as the perpetrators sit in jail, which are the arms of solitude, like Superman's Fortress of Solitude, in the Frozen wasteland of his iron, and unfeeling heart as he looks on into the world of weakness, and only sees people, who need his help as a saviour, because he is too, even though, from another planet, and a different race, can only see a reflection of himself, and so if he cannot see a reflection of himself, he tries to create one, and so with all his super powers, he tries to bring about a utopian society of Supermen, like the Nazis, the British Empire, the Holy Roman Empire, and many more. But then, what about his love, mercy, compassion, and understanding, for the weak, and is there such a thing in the Super race of men among the race of weakness? In addition, these races of Supermen reflect on the horrible crime, that they committed, and just one thing comes to mind, and that is, "I should not have done it."

It was a sign of respect that has caused another soul, their life as they look into the mirror of their own reflection, and what do they see, looking back at them in the mirror of perception? It is a murderer, someone who is dark, and has taken a life, and the truth is there is no way back from taking a life, because if you have understanding of the mathematical equation of the reflection in the mirror of perception, then you will understand when these individuals took another life, they were trying to erase their own, by killing their own reflection, in what they thought was their enemy but in truth, just reminded them of what they hated, the most in themselves, that is why I think war is madness, because all we are really doing, is eradicating our darkness, that we see in our ourselves, being reflected in our adversaries, in war, and the truth is it will never go away, because we do not understand, what we are seeing, being reflected in the mirror of life, back at us, and that is our own darkness. Therefore, the sad truth is, war will always be with us until, if we can realize, that our worst enemies are not the other man, in another foreign country but the way we see, that man in our own image, which is our own image of what we hate, and dislike in ourselves. This is called flight as we see with Superman, by creating an alter ego of our darkness, the things we do not like about ourselves, we project them onto a race, that is weaker in America during the civil rights movement, it was the Afro-Americans, hence they became the alter ego of the white race, and because the Afro-Americans could not fight back, the white Americans were able to fly, like a bird or was it a plane, no it was the race of Supermen or the race of a Superman, thus making their own laws, and justice to suite their needs, for power to sustained what they thought was the light but in truth was the darkness revealed in the light, for everyone to see for themselves, what they really were at that period of time.

But nothing really changes, because no one understands the mirror of reflection, accept for Jesus as he died on the cross, and the whole world saw, what they looked like as his body was deformed from all the beatings, being spat on, his bread ripped from his skin, because he loved the poor, the weak, and the helpless, and that he wanted them to live, and have good, and honest lives, free from wars, famines, diseases, plagues, and the most horrid ways, that these races of Supermen have killed them in his name. And so, when the famous president broke down in public as he condemned himself, by calling himself by what he saw in his enemies, the main reason why he went to war, in the first place, and that was he hated the idea, that religious men should use religion as a pretext for war, and conflict but in truth that is exactly what he did by committing many to a war, that cannot be won, simply because we are fighting our own shadows, and if you notice with a shadow you cannot touch it, or catch it, and you can only see it, while there is sun light but when it is dark, there is no reference point to behold our shadow, and so when it is completely dark, there will be no way to disguised the

If I Am Then I Must Be

shadow of our own psychotic natures in war, and so the trumpet of, 'Doomsday,' is sounded, and all gather at the table of debate but since there is no more light, we all believe that we are the light, and at one synchronized moment in time, we all press the red button, that lights up the blue sky, and turn it to red, and then the end, that we see in most parts of the world today, and is also responsible for teen-age boys' novel interest in sex, rock, in addition, roll, and video games, rather than academic studies, and the pursuit of a higher knowledge. Unfortunately, these interests are not attached, with fully-grown attitudes on the subject of wellbeing, and prolonged applauses. Statistics demonstrates that young people's testosterones accounts for one-quarter of the 12 million cases of violence and civil unrest that is reported each year. Therefore, we have to consider what we are teaching our young generation as their core set of values.

The good news is that teen-agers are young, and strong, and can always change, by getting the message. And that is social gonorrhoea, that is getting drunk, partying all night, doing drugs, and so on, just plain old civil disobedience, in most cases, among adolescent boys, has to do, is not the right way to go, and must decrease, over the next seven years or there won't be anything left. However, boys' interest in girls is now purely sexual. Compared with my generation, boyhood is more religiously built on the computer games, rock, and roll, and the fantasy drama, that is likely to have relationships with the chaotic nature of life, and so the stresses of life, wears out the young teenager, and so the girls agree with the survey statements, like there is nothing for the young to do in this country but get drunk, and have babies. Nevertheless, wait a minute; is not life what you make of it? Then why make a song, and dance, why not be like the Americans, and that is, 'to be all that you can be.' By spending your time in scholarly pursuits, and allow the boys, and girls, to both express their feelings, not as how the academic world sees British life but how they see British life in the new light of the age old scholarly pursuit of educational excellence. And let the hormones stay frozen, like Superman's heart, until they are mature enough to settle down with their rightful soul mates, and let their interest in sex not goad them toward risky, and aggressive behaviours, that leads to endless sorrows and woes.

Chapter 15

But however, if a man can produce a name or a mathematical equation of a logical consequence, to produce a proven ideology, in the theoretical school of theoretical form, that is ideas to thoughts, and then to concepts, an idea, that a thought exist, then it is so, and so hence, the theorem, the logical mathematical provability of the proposition forum of the formula, in the mathematical equation of the thought, 'If I am then I must be,' the ideology of two or more opposing ideas, that becomes thoughts, which leads to oppositions, divisions, and ultimately chaos for, 'if I am then I must be,' to be no more, hence 1, if I am, 2, then I must be.

For the foolish mind will agree, 'if I am than I am and I cannot be, because to be is not to be for if I am then I cannot be,' because omnipresence does not exist in the fallen race of Adam so I cannot be in two schools of theoretical thought concepts at the same time, just as I cannot be in England, and India at the same time, in the same spatial reference point. I am either in the light or I am either in the dark, I am either night or I am either day, I am either good or I am either evil, I am either sick or I am either well, I am either rich or I am either poor, I either believe in the existence of God through Jesus or I either believe in the non existence of God through Jesus. It is the logic of the provable form, a set of axioms, and basic assumptions, ideas, and ideology, the modern mythology of the modern Homo sapiens, the creation of the alter ego of Mary Shelly's, in her Frankenstein monster, hence known as the feminist movement, the communist movement, the a partied movement, which is an idea of ideals, accepted or proposed as true from the Latin via the mid 16th century, from the root of the Greek word theorema, 'speculation,' from theorin, 'to look at,' from theoros, the ethos of gambling, and so back to my original thought, and that is if a thing exist, then it is so, and so hence the theorem, that explains light as being a proton of a stable nuclear particle of electrical energy, an elementary particle of the baryon family, that is a component of all atomic nucei, and carries a positive charge, equal to that of the electron's negative charge. A type of the elementary particle of a subatomic particle, belonging to the group, that has undergone the strong interactions, and of change of the mass of ideas conceived in the night to the greater thoughts, expressed in the light of our limited understanding of the greater picture of the ideals of duality. In addition, so light proves energy exists in both realms of the theatre of theological time, hence the ethos of the paradox of two points existing in the same spatial reference point. Hence the concepts of night, and day existing in the same spatial coordinates as relative space, and if scientist can create in their own image, a theorem, that equates the logical existence of the concepts of light, then it is real, and in this realm of logic cannot change, if this theorem is true, then light has always existed, and will always exists, and he said, "I am that I am, I am the same yesterday, and today, and forever, I the light, that heals thee, and I change not, before Abraham your father I was, I am the Alpha and the Omega, I am the beginning and the end," and if light proven by the scientific communities of ideas, and ideals become thought in being the concept of, "if I am then I must be," proves the theorem of light, then there is no end to this voice, that echoes in the heart of ideas, and ideals, then light has always existed, and will always exists, and he said, "I am that I am, I am the same yesterday, and today, and forever, I the light that heals thee, and I change not, before Abraham your father was, I am the light, I am the Alpha, and the Omega, I am the beginning, and the end, and I am the light of the world, whoever walks in me shall not walk in the darkness." And if the scientific community can prove that light existed first, then the night, which is the alternative perception of the light, which was in the beginning, which is light slowed down to conceptual thought, thus becoming, sound, touch, taste, smell, and sight, hence the ideology of experience.

Chapter 16

It is said, through conceptual thought turned into theoretical speech that light is made up of small particles, defined as photons, hence the name given to define in the realm of experience, that is the realm of touch, sound, taste, smell, and sight of what light is, and in so defining with understanding what cannot be understood as touch, sound, taste, smell, and sight, experience cannot touch light with flesh, because it is not a solid material, experience cannot taste light, because it is not solid enough to eat, and in such has not taste that the human taste buds of the human experience can taste, experience cannot smell light, because it has no smell, that can be recognize by the human experience called smell, experience cannot see light, because it is not solid enough or more rather slow enough, that the human eyes can see with experience, and so the theorems of the concepts of light is based on an conceptual idea, and that is, 'if I am then I must be,' in its original form, which is light, and so bringing light into the concept of thought turned into theoretical ideas, and so we bring the ethos of light into the mirror of our own perceptions of the reflection of ourselves in the mirror of life personified as our myths, traditions, fables, of what we think we are in the light, and that is if, 'I am then I must be.'

Hence the darkness of our id, our hidden desires, which is the colour black reversed, becoming the colour white in the realm of experience so we now have the moral authority to say who we kill in wars, who we bless, hence the age of technical discoveries, that promotes technologies, that produces commerce, medical advances, that produces wealth but denies the poor, those who have no voice, the right to these life prolonging discoveries, while the true blackness of hearts is ignored as we watch the poor starve to death, in the developing world, and even in our nations as we tax the poor to death, to build our utopian world of darkness, personified as light, hence the reinvention of Mount Olympus, personified in the game of life, which is now the game of death as we champion the cause of, 'if I am then I must be,' and so the moral thought, which is light, becomes the expressed thought of the immoral conscious, which is black, hence what is black becomes white, and what is white becomes black, and that is we in the light of our understanding of the reflection of the blackness of our hearts became the light by which we exist, and, "In the beginning God created the heaven, and the earth.

And the earth was without form, and void; and darkness *was* upon the face of the earth, and the darkness of human understanding personified in experience of touch, taste, sound, smell, sight, form the earth in its own image, that is void of all human understanding of love thy neighbour as thyself, which is the light, and now becomes darkness hate thy neighbour personified as light, and the face of the deep blackness of the human soul experience. Moreover, the Spirit of God moved upon the face of the waters. Moreover, God said, Let there be light: and there was light. And God saw the light, that *it was* good: and God divided the light from the darkness. And God called, hence the experience of touch, smell, taste, sight, sound, light but the experience of light, became the experience of darkness of the heart of human reasoning personified as the light in the human experience, when light of the experience of touch, smell, taste, sight, sound became the experience of touch, smell, taste, sight, sound of the darkness of the human experience, hence when thought consumed the forbidden fruit, and so perception of the light of the experience of touch, smell, taste, sight, sound the ethos of inversion the reversal of the natural order of existence, and life became death, because now that thought had consumed the Apple of Knowledge of dark, and light, human reasoning came into being, and so a new consciousness was form in man, and hence it was, 'If I am then I must be,' and so immoral becomes moral, and moral became immoral, for if, 'I am then I must be,' lust became love, and love became lust, for, 'if I am then I must be,' and stealing, and killing became honor, and honor became stealing, and killing, and so is immortalized in the honored amongst the children of men. As we remember the death and forget the living. And so when the light slowed down from its original speed of 86,000 miles per second, to the speed of thought turned into theoretical speech of the conceptual theoram of experience, which is the creation of the, 'Homo sapiens,' the modern man of ideas, made thought made experience, and in so light becomes touch, sound, taste, smell, and sight of the dark void of the id of Homo sapiens psyche."

Then spake the light for the second time, again unto them, saying, "I am the light of the world: he that followeth me shall not walk in darkness but shall have the light of life." The darkness inverted as light, personified in the Pharisees therefore said, "In the beginning was the light, and the light was with the light, and the light was light. The same was in the beginning with light.

All things were made by the light; and without the light was not anything made that were made. In the light was light; and the light was the light of men. And the light shineth in darkness; and the darkness comprehended it not," then the light said, "There was a man sent from the light, whose name *was the light*. The same came for a witness, to bear witness of the light, that all *men* through the light might believe, that light is, and was, and will be forever. The light was not that light, but *was sent* to bear witness of that light." And the Pharisees said, "T*hat* we are the true light, which lighteth every man, that cometh into the world." And the light said, "The light was in the world, and the world was made by the light, and the world knew the light not, because they were the personified darkness of the world that became the personified light of the world. And the light came unto his the light, and his own the light received the light, not because they were the light." But as many as received the light, to them gave he power to become the true image of the light, even to them that believe on his name: which is the true light of the world, were born, not of blood, nor of the will of the flesh, which is the dark inverted as the light, nor of the will of the darkness in men's thoughts but of the true light of all just men's hearts.

And the light became Word, the expression light, and in so light became touch, sound, taste, smell, and sight of the light made flesh, and so dwelt among us, (and we beheld his light, the light as of the only begotten of the source of the light,) full of grace, and truth. And so the light bare witness of the light, and cried, saying, "This was the true light of whom I spake, He that cometh after me is preferred before me; for he was before me. And this is the condemnation, that light is came into the world, and men loved the light rather than light, because their deeds were good, and good from the tree of the knowledge of good, and evil, hence the inverted thought of good, and evil becoming the inverted thought of good, and good. For everyone, that doeth good hates the light, neither cometh to the light, lest his deeds should be reproved in the light, because he is the light." So the light becomes a particle, and a wave in the realm of touch, sight, sound, smell, and taste but however not only a wave, and then sometimes a particle, and so hence the children of the light took hundreds of years to accept what it is, for the light exist in the moment of ideas of conceptual thought, in the ideals of touch, taste, smell, and sound trying to be the moment, and so only existing in the moment like the famous speech of the great light, when the light asked him his name, and he said "I am that I am," he is the moment, when the moment exist, not when the moment has gone, and another begins And that moment is, in the now, and not in the past, trying to create the future light of the world by rebuilding the pass light of the past, for the future as in the famous speeches of the leaders of the light of the past, trying to create the light of the future, without considering the presence moment, where the light can only exist, and can be seen, touched, smelt, heard, and speak, 'that we will allow the utilities companies to keep prices high in the moment, where the true light is for the moment of the future light as the light in the present moment suffers as the light tries to understand the future moment, when the future moment does not exist in the present moment, and the law of the moment is governed by the law of time in experience, the old saying, 'you only live once,' which is in the present moment, where you are, and experience touch, taste, smell, sound, and sight in that present moment of time,' and the present light, that exist in the moment is extinguished, by having to make hard choices on whether to feed themselves or keep themselves warm, until the moment of the future comes where the light of the modern man, the moral man, which is the light as he evolves into the Homo sapiens, from the Homo Erectus exist, and since the future moment is in the future, it never comes, because the now is the present moment, that exist in the present, while the future moment is yet to come, and when the future moment comes, it is the present moment,' Hence Winston Churchill strategy in winning World War II as in his famous speech rephrase in the ideology of common sense, "In order to know your future you must understand your past."

So when the humanist, the future light to come makes statements, that there is no light, they are right, for the light does not exist in the past, hence the theorem of evolution, nor does he exist in the future, where Utopia is found, the Heavenly Jerusalem of the light of the heart of modern man, hence the moral man, the light of the world, because the light is, 'I am that I am,' and is in this moment of time, with those who live, and see in this is moment of time. And the light, that exist in the past trying to create the future is now shaped in the ideology of the scientific community, an electromagnetic wave like radio waves, microwaves, X rays, and so on, and they begin, when electric charges goes back, and forth, hence two in one concept of I am I must be having, both an electric – field, and a magnetic field, moving together, and like photons, they move in a straight line. But however is subject to a variety of forms, based on the frequency of the electrometric wave, thus producing different kinds of waves, hence radio waves, being of a very low frequency, whereas the microwaves, then infrared light, and then the visible spectrum formed in different colours of the rainbow.

If I Am Then I Must Be

Chapter 17

And as no one will love us so we fantasize as we remunerate on our broken hearts, by how we are portrayed by educated men, and as I remunerate in my lonely world, I am King Arthur Smith, and the Duke of Cornwall Smith, and Morgana Smith, and Igrayne Smith, and more, for in my lonely world of my imagination, I am who I want to be, and not what I have been labeled by Doctors, and scientists, and meanwhile, the Duke of Cornwall Smith is killed during his assault, and sensing her father's death.

Believing her husband to return home, Igrayne Smith makes love to an aggressive Uther Smith, while a devastated Morgana Smith sees past to a son, Arthur Smith. Upon seeing his child, Uther Smith speaks of creating peace, and staying with Igrayne Smith. Much to Igrayne's Smith despair, Merlin Smith later arrives, and reminds Uther Smith of the oath he took, and takes baby Arthur Smith. Uther Smith pursues Merlin Smith, and is later ambushed by the remaining loyal Cornwall Smith's knights, who were also after Excalibur Smith. He is mortally wounded, in the forest but not before thrusting the sword Smith into a large nearby stone.

Witnessing this, Merlin Smith exclaims that, "he who draws the sword Smith from the stone, he shall be King Smith." Years later, Sir Ector Smith, and his sons Kay Smith, and Arthur Smith attend a jousting tournament, to win a chance to draw Excalibur Smith, from the stone. The best knights Smith in the land gather to compete and Leondegrance Smith is the victor but fails to pull the sword from its stone prison Smith. Arthur Smith, now Kay's Smith squire, forgets Kay's Smith sword in a tent, and returns only to discover, that it has been stolen. While pursuing the thief, Arthur Smith stumbles by the stone in which the Excalibur Smith is embedded. By sheer fate, and destiny, the sword Smith calls to him and Arthur Smith draws it from the stone. Once news arrived of the sword Smith's release, the tournament crowd gather around him. Sir Ector Smith commands Arthur Smith to put it back, and after a failed attempt by a sceptical Uyrens Smith, Arthur Smith easily draws the sword from the stone once more. Merlin Smith then appears, revealing to Arthur Smith, that he is the son of Uther Smith, and Igrayne Smith, hence by

birthright; he is the rightful King Smith of the land. Not all accept
Arthur Smith's kingship. As the knights Smith argue, a confused
Arthur Smith flees into the forest pursuing Merlin Smith. He later
explains Arthur Smith's destiny, telling the boy Smith, that he and
the land are one. Overwhelmed, Arthur Smith slips off into sleep.
The next morning, Merlin Smith tells him, that his enemies are
laying siege to the castle of one of Arthur Smith main supporters,
Leondegrance Smith. Rallying the other knights Smith loyal to him,
Arthur Smith leads a counter-assault, and repels the attacker
Smith's. The battle Smith ends when Arthur Smith asks for Sir
Uryens Smith's faith in Arthur Smith's newfound kingship.

Uryens Smith is insulted at swearing faith to a squire Smith. Arthur
Smith realizing what he says is true, gives Excalibur Smith to him to
proclaim Arthur Smith, a knight. Tempted to take the sword for
himself, Uryens Smith hesitates, but after seeing Arthur Smith's
humility and courage in battle, grants his request. Afterwards,
Arthur Smith later meets Leondegrance Smith's daughter
Guenevere Smith, who narrowly avoids a kiss from Arthur Smith,
while she helps mend his wounds, Later, Arthur Smith, and his
knights Smith encounter a brilliant, and self-proclaimed undefeated
knight Smith named Lancelot Smith. In search of a king Smith,
worthy of his sword, Lancelot Smith will allow none to pass a
bridge, until he is defeated in single combat. After besting all of
Arthur Smith's knights, Arthur Smith himself engages Lancelot
Smith in a joust.

An enraged Arthur Smith refuses to accept Lancelot Smith besting
him, and challenges Lancelot Smith in a duel to the death Smith.
The two combatants fight brings them near a nearby lake. Lancelot
Smith is surprisingly fast and agile striking at will on the furious
and unbalanced Arthur Smith. Laying on the rocks in defeat, Arthur
Smith summons Excalibur Smith's power. The, 'Sword Smith of
Power,' hums with magic, and cuts through Lancelot Smith's spear,
piercing his armour, and knocking him unconscious but breaking the
sword in half, in the process. A devastated and shameful Arthur
Smith confesses to Merlin Smith, that in his rage he abused the
sword's power, to serve his own vanity. Arthur Smith throws what
is left of the sword into the nearby body of water but, upon his
words of contrition, the, 'Lady of the Lake Smith,' shows herself,

and offers a restored Excalibur Smith to the king Smith. Realizing his error, Arthur Smith quietly vows never to abuse the sword's power again.

Lancelot Smith awakens, and realized he was finally bested, swears fearfully to Arthur Smith. After a series of battles, Arthur Smith, and his knights Smith unify the land. He decides to create a Round Table Smith, and builds his castle, Camelot Smith. Arthur Smith ultimately marries Guenevere Smith but upon escorting her to the wedding, Lancelot Smith falls deeply in love with her. Arthur Smith's half-sister, Morgana Smith, a budding sorceress, becomes apprenticed to Merlin Smith, in hopes of learning the Charm of Making from him. Time passes and Lancelot Smith, the greatest of the knights, is often inexplicably absent from the Round Table, seeking refuge deep in the forest, in order to brood. One day while sleeping in the forest, Lancelot Smith encounters a peasant boy named Percival Smith, who aspires to become a knight Smith, and impresses Lancelot Smith with his resiliency. Lancelot Smith guides him back to Camelot Smith, where Percival Smith, later becomes his squire. Though the king Smith's champion, Lancelot Smith's forbidden love for Guenevere Smith keeps him away from Camelot Smith. One evening, Sir Gawain Smith, under the corruption of Morgana Smith, openly accuses both knight, and queen of adultery at the Round Table. Since he is King Smith, Arthur Smith decrees, that he must be the judge, and that Lancelot Smith must defend Guenevere Smith's honour, in a duel against Gawain Smith. In a nightmare duel with himself, Lancelot Smith pierces himself, with his own sword, in order to purge himself of his love for Guenevere Smith. As the crowd gather for the duel, Lancelot Smith is nowhere to be seen. A disappointed Arthur Smith looks upon all of his knights Smith, and not one volunteer to challenge Gawain Smith, except the squire, Percival Smith.

In duress, and to the shock of the crowd, Arthur Smith hastily knights, Percival Smith. Lancelot Smith finally arrives, and despite his injuries, manages to defeat Gawain Smith, and have him withdraw his accusation. The duel is too much for Lancelot Smith, and he collapses, close to death. Arthur Smith implores Merlin Smith, to bring him back, whatever the cost, and so Merlin Smith does, placing Guenevere Smith's hand on Lancelot Smith's heart, giving him will to live. Ultimately, Guenevere Smith, realizing her love for Lancelot Smith, rides out into the forest, and the two consummate their love. A heartbroken Arthur Smith, realizing the two people he loved most in the world, have betrayed him, finds Guenevere Smith, and Lancelot Smith asleep together in the forest. Meanwhile, Merlin guides Morgana, to his secret lair intending on luring Morgana into a trap, which is showing signs of hostility towards her half-brother Arthur Smith. In the forest, Arthur Smith thrusts Excalibur Smith between the sleeping couple, and because of his magical link with the Dragon, and Earth, Merlin Smith is instantly impaled by the magical sword also. Seeing a weakened Merlin Smith, Morgana Smith seizes the opportunity to trap him, in crystal with the Charm of Making.

Morgana Smith, (like Uther Smith to Igrayne Smith,) then takes the form of Guenevere Smith, and seduces Arthur Smith, into making love to her. She later bears a son named Mordred Smith, and what you sow you reap in another generation, protects him with the magic, that no man-made weapon can kill him. On awakening to the sight of Excalibur Smith, Lancelot Smith cries, "The King Smith without a sword, the land without a King Smith," and flees, in shame as Guenevere Smith lays there weeping. Time passes, and the land is stricken with famine, and sickness, and a broken Arthur Smith sends his knights Smith on a quest for the Holy Grail, believing the land will prosper with the finding. More years pass, and many knights Smith die on the quest, while some are the walking dead; bewitched by Morgana Smith, to serve her and her son. Stopping by a lake for water, Percival Smith witnesses Mordred Smith viciously murdering Uryens Smith. In his dying breath, Uryens Smith tells Percival Smith, that he is the last of the quest knights Smith, and that he must continue his search.

Tricked by Mordred Smith, and Morgana Smith, Percival Smith manages to escape but not before, he dreams of obtaining the grail. Wandering aimlessly, Percival Smith encounters a fat, bearded, and bitter Lancelot Smith, preaching to his followers of the failures of the kingdom. Recognizing Lancelot Smith, Percival Smith tries to tell him that he is still needed by Arthur, but with the help of his followers, Lancelot Smith pushes Percival Smith into a river. Rising out of the river, Percival Smith, having lost his armour, has a vision of the Grail, and a mysterious figure who asks, "Who am I?" and, "What is my secret?" Percival Smith realizes, that the figure is King Arthur Smith, and his secret is, that he, and the land are one. Answering the riddle, he attains the Grail. Arthur Smith drinks from it, and is revitalized. Realizing, that now is his time to truly be king, Arthur Smith, and his few remaining knights Smith ride to war against Mordred Smith, and Morgana Smith. The barren land blooms, with life as they pass, reborn with its King Smith. Realizing Guenevere Smith joined a nunnery, Arthur Smith pays a visit to her convent, where they reconcile. She reveals Excalibur Smith to him, having kept it safe, since the day she fled. Most of the land's nobles have rallied to Mordred Smith, and Morgana Smith. In despair, Arthur Smith calls to Merlin Smith, and strikes a monolith in frustration, unknowingly awakening the wizard Smith from his enchanted slumber. Though still imprisoned in crystal, Merlin Smith appears to Morgana Smith in dream, and tricks her into calling the dragon, and uttering the Charm of Making, creating a thick fog of the dragon's breath.

Her magically endowed youth dissolves much to the dismay of her son Mordred Smith as he strangles her to death in disgust. With the help of Merlin Smith, Arthur Smith, and his jolly knights survive using Morgana Smith's mist to their advantage, to hide their small numbers but are soon overwhelmed. Out of the fog arrives Lancelot Smith, who joins the fray, and turns the tide of the battle. After disposing of the remaining enemies, Lancelot Smith falls to the ground from the old wound that never healed. Arthur Smith, and Lancelot Smith reconcile, and Lancelot Smith dies with Arthur Smith's approval, that he was the Round Table's greatest knight. A distraught Arthur Smith turns to find Mordred Smith, ready to embrace his father with a spear. Percival Smith offers to fight but Arthur Smith, realizing Mordred Smith was his sin, stands to face his son. Mordred Smith lunges forward with his weapon, and pierces Arthur Smith but the determined King Smith pulls the spear, and his son, closer to him, and stabs Mordred Smith with the enchanted blade of Excalibur Smith, killing him. Knowing his time has come, Arthur Smith commands Percival Smith to throw Excalibur Smith in a pool of calm water, where it is caught by the glimmering scale-clad hand of the, 'Lady of the Lake Smith,' When Percival Smith returns, he witnesses Arthur Smith's body on a ship sailing away. The king Smith is attended by three formally posed ladies clad in white, sailing into the setting sun toward the Isle of Avalon.

If I Am Then I Must Be

Chapter 18

It was a great big culture shock to my system to find out that I was black, and in America, no one likes black people unless they were successful. But I was a poor black man, who had nothing to show for my life. I saw how some white men, lusted after the black women especially, if they were voluptuous, with big breast, and a firm round bottom, and nice strong leg. But however, the white parasites, but not all were so, just those, that I had encountered, would feast of all my knowledge of the human condition but yet they treated me like I had a human conditional disease, that was only approachable, when I had some brilliant concept for them to feed on. I remembered how my photography teacher would act like a dog in heat at Patricia who was in his class.

However, Patricia knew how to tease men, to get what she wanted, and she would not to give it up easy as most young black American women did, and not the older generation of Afro American models, in fact it reminded me of the pop song titled, 'suicidal,' and how most young black women were as they over acted sexually, and they would used every trick in the book to get their men into bed as they gloat over their victories as dysphasia being difficult to understand as sexually heighten young women, which they had been program from the days of slavery until now. When in Africa the modern man the Homo sapiens went into that once great spiritual country, and murdered, raped, and destroyed a whole continent? Then when the black woman had enough of whoring they look for a, 'Mr. Reed,' the backbone of the fantastic four, someone who is shy, and has worked hard, and then they used what they have learnt, while whoring on their backs, to trap them into being their pure husbands so that they can have their cake, and eat too. Patricia was like that with me.

A dark skinned woman who fit the criteria of a voluptuous black woman. She was sensual in all her ways. She wore bright red lipstick to seduce her prey as Cleopatra did to entice Mark Anthony, to ravish her like a hungry wild animal in search of food, knowing, that the first to think to destroy an empire, and the Holy Roman Empire at that was to create jealousy, between to powerful forces.

Now we call it racism but first it is recorded in the bed as Cleopatra seduced her prey as she hypnotized him by her big golden brown breast, and her seductive legs, and her golden silk body the Phoenix reborn, which drove him mad, that he would fight against Rome, for a piece of ass, and that was all it was. But I knew the technique very well. I knew that some higher force of men, had destroyed the black female, and then removed the dignity from the black male species so that they could use the black woman as whore, thus enjoying all the pain, and suffering, when virtuous black, who strove so hard to build their careers, and when they had reached the top, there were no decent black men to fend for them in marriage, and it would break these virtuous black women hearts', and so they would curse the God Jesus who created them in their heart's, not knowing it was the desire of those who think they hold the power of the nations through wars, death, and destruction, calling one race, a bunch of terrorist, because they see, and know how the other side works, and that is to destroy everything, that they do not understand, by murdering them, such as innocent babies, women, and even their men saying, that if we don't do this they will kill us.

Instead of developing true human qualities, and that is to sit down at the table of debate, and reason our differences, and not kill each other, for a piece of mental, which was more important, than the holy commandment Jehovah gave to man, 'Thou shalt not kill,' and now many kill in his name, such as the crusades, the witch trials, honour killings, and so on. In addition, I just stopped for a moment as in my rumination got out of control, and I said to myself, "And I have been labelled by these people as mad but yet I do not kill my fellow man in gas chambers, calling this an act of God that is called Jesus who many believe in including me. But I am sure if he had as I do believe created life, then why would he sanction the arrogance of men mostly Governments, to take it for an ideal, that they are acting on his behalf?"

She dressed in loose fitting clothes so that you would be teased by her, not showing of her delicious figure. There was a competition between my photography teacher, and another black student as to which one she would sleep with but her eyes were on me. She knew that I was shy, and would make a good father, to her children. Patricia was looking to breed her kind into the world, and she used every trick in the book to get my attention. In the darkroom, she would hold my hand gently, and lead me around the darkroom as she tried to seduce me, in the darkness of her soul, which was very corrupt, with the desire to emulate her great, great grandmother, the African queen Cleopatra, her ancient ancestral spirit. Saying things to encourage my ego such as, "You are a big strong man." I must admit, that I loved the way that she spoke to me. My teacher was jealous of me, and so called me a clot in class, in front of all the students, because I did not get my printing right. He wanted to fail me, because Patricia wanted me, and not him. But Julia was a strong African American woman, who did not sell her soul to Saturn, and she had the dignity of her ancestor, and she fought like they did, and it cost many of them their lives, against the darkness of man's inhumanity to each other, based on the colour of their skin, who worked in the registrar office, that took a shine to me, and went after my teacher for the grade, that I so richly deserved. Julia knew she would go to fight him, because she knew he was a racist that did not like to see black people succeed. In fact, most white teachers in the school were like that.

Chapter 19

Anger flared up in me as I stood at the bus stop, on that cold and bitter winter night, for a bus, to take me home. I was upset at the way evil people just used me, and corrupted the purity, that was in me. Nevertheless, I had no way to strike out or anyone to confide in, because I was a bitter young man, and I had closed myself off, from the world, because of the child abuse, that had shaped my life. Even to this day, I will not trust anyone, unless they proved themselves to me, and that is if they are like me. As the clock struck six, the bus pulled into the bus station, and I got on. A white woman sat next to me.

She tried to make conversation with me but I was not having any of it. I just sat there, and listened to her. Nevertheless, on the inside I was being eaten away, by the insects of my past. I would not dear open my mouth, not being in control of my thoughts; I did not know what would come out. All the hate, that I had for myself, reflected back in those who I would meet, day to day, in America, that was hidden in my heart, and would come to the surface so I thought but in reality, my an ancestral father, the father of lies, that is Saturn was trying to create another Hitler, who destroyed half the world, because his father never told him, that he loved him. Therefore, he reflected his shame, and anger of his father, and his failings of his father, into the Jewish race, and built in him, the hatred to be an Antichrist, and was hidden in his heart, and would come to the surface, when he was reminded of his experience, with them.

I laughed, and joked with her but I was careful, in what I was saying, while all the time loathing her, because she had influence in the world, and I did not. "It is a cold day isn't it?" she said, in a happy go lucky way, I tried to hide my discomfort at the question she asked me, and replied, "The summers are too hot, and the winters are too cold," she noticed, that my accent was different, and asked me where I was from, "I am from England, I have lived here for nine years." "That's great, my grandparents are from Italy," she said enthusiastically, "I have noticed, that most art in the north has a European flavour," I said, she agreed with me, "Oh this is my stop," she said abruptly. Then she said she replied, "It was nice meeting you," I said nothing, and looked backed a way back, into this fantasy world, where I am king. I looked out the window of the bus as she left. She was shocked, that we had a good conversation, and I would not even say goodbye, to her but I understood what a whore really was, and that whether it is man or a woman, they feed on someone's goodness, just to sleep with them, just to feel how it feels like, in sexual union, which ruins a lot of good people, because now it is based on lust, and not spiritual love, which proceeds from our true divine natures, when Jehovah created man Adam, and his wife Eve, in the, 'Garden of Eden.' Some men would just go to college, and get certificates of honour, among men so that they can get a better piece of ass, whether they are black or white, and the women would go along with this concept, because it felt like true love, which in fact was death, because as my true spiritual father had taught me, what seems light, behind it is very dark, and what seems very dark, behind it is much light, and that is the secret to the life of Jesus on the earth, two thousand years ago, as it is written in Isaiah 52, and 53. Jesus looked like something out of a horror movie but that was the door of his house the Father's heart, which had to be guarded from being hurt, just like his Holy Spirit, when he had to destroy Israel, in the wilderness, to protect his conscience, from being emotionally damaged, that he could not accurately perform his function, to save man from hell, in their own conscience, which led the human race into the second, the spiritual form of what is called a black hole but in the earth not in space.

I could not wait for the next two stops to come, because I knew how the rest of my day would go, even before the bus pulled into the stop. I was at the door, waiting to exit the bus. As the bus stopped, at my bus stop, I quickly got off, and then I walked down the street, and turned into my road. Before I reached my apartment, I had my key in my hand. As I pushed the key, into the key hole, and turned the key, and I go into the house, and because I was poor, I could only afford a room in a house, where I had to share the bathroom, and a kitchen. I eagerly made my way to my room, I took off my coat, and then opened my room door, and I had just bought the new, 'Tears for Fears,' album, and my favourite song was called, 'Songs from the Big Chair.' Since they did not have CD players, in those days so, I would rewind the cassette, and crank up the volume as loud as it would go. Then I would pretend that, I had a twin brother, who was evil, and that my twin brother was the leader of a very powerful army, that was bent on destroying, the world through war, and that I was a general of the American forces, and I was sailing to confront my brother in war. I would dance around the room, in my mad little world completely, consumed by this fantasy, until I got bored of reliving the fights, that me, and my real brother, had as he was bigger than me, and bullied me, all the time, and out of his jealousy for me. And the truth was, until now I did not know the depths of my pain, and how hurt I really was, from the child abuse, growing up, in a dysfunctional family, and how the beatings, and other disappointments controlled my life, until now, because now I am free to be who I want to be, and not what my ancestral spirits were trying to create in me, which was their host, for all their dark arts, and I would, then turn on the television, and watch the television for the rest of the night.

Chapter 20

Because I did not have a father figure, I had to learn about life, and evil men on my own, this promoted my mental illness, to a new high. I remembered John Mark, a Haitian that I met in Boston Massachusetts. He was very quiet, when we first met. I met him through Lester Godwine, a psychopathic liar, that I had worked with at, 'Store 24,' one of a chain of stores that opened for 24 hours a day, in Boston. Lester also got me fired, from my job, which I loved, because it allowed me to study during the day. Lester told his boss, that he tried to stop some teenagers from stealing some food from the store, and that I never helped him.

Even though it was the management policy, not to stop thieves from stealing in the store, this manager was young, and an egotist, and he wanted self-glory. So he made his own rules, and because I was shy, and bitter inside at the abuse, that happened to me I was very negative towards this boss. In addition, that was the main reason why Bill fired me. It was not until I met his girlfriend that is John Mark, of course; that he saw that I was gullible, and could easily be manipulated but that was because of the mental mask, my illness had placed on me. Lester pretended to be a black belt in karate but he was an unusual black belt, because he could not even do the splits, and because I believed him, Lester said that he would train me for twenty-five dollars a session. Since I had no experience at these sorts of things I fell for it. It was after we had finished our training session, that John Mark walks into the flat, where Lester would train me, with his girlfriend, soon to be his wife. Lester introduced them to me. Susan and I got on well, while John Mark watched, and studied his prey. John Mark was known in the music world as a bad musician, who tried to use the other members of the band, that he would bring together but as usual they would wise up to what he was doing, and leave, and John Mark would be back at stage one, in trying to get his plan of world dominance into being. Nevertheless, this was different, this time he felt that he would try to use me to build his evil empire, because he knew that I had a problem with being assertive. Susan began to talk about politics, and the human condition. In addition, I began to share my knowledge of the subject. After we had tired each other out Susan excitedly said,

"This is the kind of friend, that I wish you would hang around with," Susan was more like mother to John, and John would pretend to be responsive to her. However, the real reason, that he wanted her was, because he felt, that she was also gullible, and he could use her for money, because she came from a middle class family. John Mark, like a wolf, became very friendly with me but I was feeling alone, because I had no other friends.

I thought that I could be a friend to John Mark, a sort of mother figure but that was far from the truth, John Mark had other ideas. Through my experiences, that almost cost me everything, my opponents were better equipping for the battle that we always fought against each other, than I was. I had to learn how to survive, and by the sacrifices, that I made, and so I overcame them, even though I was bitter, and filled with pain. I overcame that bitterness, and pain, and matured, and healed from all the wounds that I inflicted upon myself. I was more alive to the darkness that was sin in my life, when I was young; now the light was shinning brightly, and getting brighter, in this world of mines. My vision had grown in those days, I saw through a dark glass, and what I saw was, that I had been robbed of the beauty of my innocence, that I was a beautiful flower, that had not received any rain for many seasons, and I had shrivelled up, and began to die. However, I was not dead. I still clanged to life, because my hope was not dead, a hope to live dependably from any influences, that my damaged character had created. Saturn's character engulfing me, into someone else's world of darkness, I did not want to die for someone else's belief system, I wanted to live my own life, even though I had no clue to what it entailed. I wanted, after I had died, and stood at the judgment seat of Christ, to say that I lived for my own beliefs, shaped on my own belief, that were associated with truth. Not on someone else's, value system that had caused millions to die, without hope, and without any decision at all. Many lived their lives, not living their dreams, and did without realizing, that they have not lived. It might be a simple dream as to see most of the world; instead they are trapped, in a hopeless life.

If I Am Then I Must Be

Chapter 21

People come in all shapes, and sizes, with obvious differences, in abilities, and appearances. There are many, 'faces of Man,' found throughout the world. Yet, although the faces are different, the genetic structure, the DNA, is not as different as most people believe. Over 99% of the DNA, in all people is identical. This is not an accident. Most of the proteins that carry out the biochemical functions of a human body are made exactly the same, from one person to the next. The remaining one percent, however, accounts for people's diversity. It can also be used as a tool, to determine how genetically related people are, this sameness has been of great interest to scientists, ever since the discovery of DNA, and its function in the inherit patterns.

These scientists thought, that perhaps the study of DNA could provide essential clues, in the long-standing quest for an understanding of the evolution of Homo sapiens, and the units of abnormal cells are working out the fundamentals of the directives of every normal living activities contained in our physic selves, now called by the science community, 'parapsychology,' the study of the fallen man, and his ways of life as Charles Darwin would put it, 'the survival of the fittest.' We now call, that study, the story of the modern man or more to the point the Homo sapiens species. All that is needed to direct their system within the chemical from all organisms, that made up the chemicals of the physically organic components of our own perceptions, in the mirror of our own reflection of what we think we see in others but really is what we see in ourselves, because others only reflects our desires, hopes, and nightmares, particularly of the arrangement of the bases of the DNA strands, the order, that spells out one exact instructions, that is required to create a particular organism with itself of its own unique traits of DNA, in the human genome is arranged into 24 distinct chromosomes molecules, that range in length from 50 million to 250 million base pairs. We assumed what can be detected by microscopic examination; however most changes in DNA, are physically separate from about a few types of major chromosomal abnormalities, more subtle, and require a closer analysis of the DNA molecule, to find perhaps a single based difference. In 1979, a new specie of life is become from the realm of nothing exiting she is called a girl, and is identified by the satirist, including those in the mental health profession Doctor. Dr. Bean, and her guardian, her mother chose her to bear Saturn's son during, the last hour, on the 19th October 1964, thanks to a symbol, a star as it travelled, quite close to the earth. As she is being born, a nurse names him, 'Horace James Barrocks,' later to be known as, 'Smith,' it was a surprised to all the satirists, because they wanted a girl but however, came forth from the mother womb's was a beautiful boy, that as he grew older, they tried to turn into a girl, first by having him sodomized, at that age of ten, by two black gay catholic priests, and then with mind control, by putting subliminal messages, into his mind, that having relations with both men, and women with male body parts was ok. Which I knew was wrong for me, and so he followed his higher conscience, and never gave into these different mind controlling thoughts as so many did, before and will after him. The priest in the Vatican witnessed the star as it whizzed by the earth, and described it as the, 'Eye of God,' that would usher in the age of enlightenment for all mankind, 'the Age of Aquarius,' the age without human compassion but however, I chose human compassion, and not Saturn, which was a great problem to the satirist for it heralding the birth of the one chosen to be the son of God, however not the perfect son of God but nevertheless a son of God, who would follow the father Saturn wherever he went.

And as I began to remunerate in my mad world of dark images, and vain ideas, the molecules to find the single based differences, those are the genes, that specifically causes madness of the sequences of an abnormal life, and existence based, that encoded instruction on how to make what is normally like the abnormal, the genes comprise of only about 2% of the human scientist knowledge of schizophrenia, the remainder consists of non understandable coding regionally found in the id of the psyche formally known as, 'The Oedipus Rex. Complex,' those functions may include providing the chromosomal of madness of the fallen mind as it began to erupt, like the Green Hulk as I enquired into my mad world to make sense of the sane world, a world where little babies are being murdered in the womb, where Politicians are taking bribes, mothers are watching all their hopes, and dreams dashed to pieces on the rock of hard men as Politicians send their children, who they raised to obey the law of the land, not to kill, not to steal as the Politicians as I have already said send them to fight in wars, calling them conflicts, and the theatre of war as if murdering each other for a piece of dirt, is entertainment like Shakespeare, and the Globe theatre. As the Politicians act out their fantasies of being the Gods on Mount Olympus as they battle in the realm of the Titians, exterminating all opposition to their end time games, and that is to create an utopian society as we see in most Science fiction dramas included, is the missing copies of the rejoining of the common goal of every man, and woman, and child, and that is peace on earth to every single human being, that is alive, hence the ideology of the Human Rights Courts in Cedex Europe. Nevertheless, if we are sending our young men to kill, in the name of freedom, then why have a court of Human Rights? For whose human rights are they protecting? Is not all life sacred, do not all mothers weep for their dead babies; do not all fathers grieve in anger for their lost children? Then why single out one specific group of people for special treatment, when all in the three-course meal, in the theatre of war suffers, the same, and none is different.

Therefore, in my mad little world, where no one cares about me, I try to fathom the mysteries of this creation, from the dead the Frankenstein, the fictional character of Mary Shelly's alter ego like Clark Kent, being Superman alter ego called the modern man, now known as the Homo sapiens, derived from the teaching of Charles Darwin evolution of the origin of species as we see what this species has evolved into as we count the death toll in World War 1 and World War 2, considering all Soviet casualties as European, and all European colonial forces as European as well.

Civilian deaths	**47'661,800**
Military Deaths	**25,280,100**
Total deaths	**72,941,900**

Chapter 22

The constellation of all human beings is in a cell that is called life. Unlike the relatively unchanging facts of wars, famines, and diseases, that destroys our wellbeing, the dynamic changes in our living environments, such as, when many Europeans colonialized other more primitive continents, and in so caught diseases, that almost killed them off, or brought diseases, that almost killed of the indigent population of that era, from minute to minute, in response to tens of thousands of intra- basaltic rockets of man's own greed, and his animalistic nature, to conquer, control so that he is known as a God among men. Each chromosome contains many ideals, and rationalities, and different opinions, that leads always to conflict, the basic physical, and functional units of heredity nature as in the jungle of humanism, that the strongest survives, and the weak is consumed into the matrix of the human evolution process of creating a utopian world, where no one feels differently, hurt, hungers, and dies, the structural integrity, and regulations of where, when, and in what quantity human grace, which is the same word for pride, and arrogance as one famous leader said in reference to another leader saying, that he has made the rich richer, and the poor poorer, and in his little world, he replies, "At least I am the good Samaritan that does not walk by on the other side." Hence, his ego comes into play, and so a chemical called euphoric protein is made, formerly known as testosterone. The human norm, that causes wars, famines, diseases, and then finally leads to death, to be remembered no more, an estimated to container of about 30,000 to 40,000 billion genes of testosterone in every human being on the face of this planet.

Although the genes of the human norm, that causes wars, famines, diseases, and then finally leads to death, to be remembered no more, an estimated container of about 30,000 to 40,000 billion genes of testosterone gets, a lot of attention as we see in the movies, that are made, and the plays, and poems, that are written about such tragic circumstances, like those poor children, that we all watched dying of cancer, on dying television, and just image to get the well deserved dignity for their families, and remember it was their grandfathers, and grandmothers, who sacrificed their lives, on the battlefield of change to uphold the right to choose a free, and developing society as to be forced to choose a editorship run by a tyrant, who's main purpose in government was to seek revenge on his father as he murdered, and killed all those who reminded him of his own reflection of how hideous he had became, and as he struck out at the weak, he was in truth trying to erase himself, from his own conscience as he is tortured in the great mighty prison, in the abyss of our disgust at what we as civilized people can do in times of great stress, and woe.

And yet their grandparents, fought in two world wars, and to get what these great men, and women of ancient times fought for, for their grandchildren, these poor, dying, lonely children have to sell their stories of their fears of the unknown, their regrets of not being there for their lovely children's children, and their never ending heart ache of being separated from their true love, the only people who accepted them for who they were, and not for what they could do for the image of the Beast. Hence, the image of commerce gone to seed, and so we call ourselves civilized nations of God fearing people but lets us look at our own hearts, and how we portray our dark secrets, that we should do in secret as light, and when all the world see the light as Hitler did what would they say, would it not be the same as Hitler did, and that is try to erase the darkness, in the his own reflection in humanity, by wiping out half the world, and if this is so, then what would happen if all nations tried to erase the darkness of their own souls as it is reflected in other races, and nations, and so the great slogan is pronounced from on high, and that is we are the light, and so they press the red button to destroy the darkness of their own souls, and those who they see as the darkness of their own souls, in the light of those who see the darkness of their own souls, in the darkness of the light of their adversary pronounced from the mountain tops, that we are the light, and so they press the red button to erase the darkness of their own souls as they see the horrid deformity of their own natures, in the mirror of the reflection of their own perceptions of themselves, in their enemies, and so we have it, 'Doomsday,' has arrived, and we all see in the light, that is the light of complete nuclear war all over the world at the same time. "And I saw in the right hand of him that sat on the throne a book written within and on the back side, sealed with seven seals. In addition, I saw a strong angel proclaiming with a loud voice, "Who is worthy to open the book, and to loose the seals thereof?" In addition, no man in heaven, or in earth, neither under the earth, was able to open the book, neither to look thereon. In addition, I wept much, because no man was found worthy to open, and to read the book, neither to look thereon. And one of the elders saith unto me, "Weep not: behold, the Lion of the tribe of Judah, the Root of David, hath prevailed to open the book, and to loose the seven seals thereof." And I beheld, and, lo, in the midst of the throne, and of the four beasts, and in the midst of the elders, stood a Lamb as it had been slain, having seven horns, and seven eyes, which are the seven Spirits of God sent forth into all the earth. And he came, and took the book out of the right hand of him, that sat upon the throne. And when he had taken the book, the four beasts, and four, *and* twenty elders fell down before the Lamb, having every one of them harps, and golden vials full of odours, which are the prayers of saints. And they sung a new song, saying, Thou art worthy to take the book, and to open the seals thereof: for thou was slain, and hast redeemed us to God by thy blood out of every kindred, and tongue, and people, and nation; and hast made us unto our God kings, and priests: and we shall reign on the earth. And I beheld, and I heard the voice of many angels round about the throne, and the beasts, and the elders: and the number of them was ten thousand times ten thousand, and thousands of thousands; saying with a loud voice, Worthy is the Lamb, that was slain to receive power, and riches, and wisdom, and strength, and honour, and glory, and blessing.

And every creature, which is in heaven, and on the earth, and under the earth, and such as are in the sea, and all, that are in them, heard I saying, Blessing, and honour, and glory, and power, *be* unto him that sitteth upon the throne, and unto the Lamb for ever, and ever. And the four beasts said, Amen. And the four and twenty elders fell down, and worshipped him, that lives for ever, and ever. And I saw when the Lamb opened one of the seals, and I heard as it were the noise of thunder, one of the four beasts saying, "Come and see." And I saw, and behold a white horse: and he that sat on him had a bow; and a crown was given unto him: and he went forth conquering, and to conquer. And when he had opened the second seal, I heard the second beast say, "Come and see." And there went out another horse that *was* red: and *power* was given to him, that sat thereon to take peace from the earth, and that they should kill one another: and there was given unto him a great sword. And when he had opened the third seal, I heard the third beast say, "Come and see." And I beheld, and lo a black horse; and he, that sat on him, had a pair of balances in his hand. And I heard a voice in the midst of the four beasts say, "A measure of wheat for a penny, and three measures of barley for a penny; and *see* thou hurt not the oil and the wine." And when he had opened the fourth seal, I heard the voice of the fourth beast say, "Come and see." And I looked, and behold a pale horse: and his name that sat on him was Death, and Hell followed with him. And power was given unto them, over the fourth part of the earth, to kill with sword, and with hunger, and with death, and with the beasts of the earth. And when he had opened the fifth seal, I saw under the altar the souls of them that were slain for the word of God, and for the testimony, which they held: and they cried with a loud voice, saying, "How long, O Lord, holy and true, dost thou not judge and avenge our blood on them that dwell on the earth?" And white robes were given unto every one of them; and it was said unto them, that they should rest yet for a little season, until their fellow servants also, and their brethren, that should be killed as they *were,* should be fulfilled.

And I beheld, when he had opened the sixth seal, and, lo, there was a great earthquake; and the sun became black as sackcloth of hair, and the moon became as blood; and the stars of heaven fell unto the earth, even as a fig tree casteth her untimely figs, when she is shaken of a mighty wind. And the heaven departed as a scroll when it is rolled together; and every mountain, and island were moved out of their places. And the kings of the earth, and the great men, and the rich men, and the chief captains, and the mighty men, and every bondman, and every free man, hid themselves in the dens, and in the rocks of the mountains; and said to the mountains, and rocks, "Fall on us, and hide us from the face of him that sitteth on the throne, and from the wrath of the Lamb: for the great day of his wrath is come; and who shall be able to stand?" And after these things, I saw four angels standing on the four corners of the earth, holding the four winds of the earth, that the wind should not blow on the earth, nor on the sea, nor on any tree. And I saw another angel ascending from the east, having the seal of the living God: and he cried with a loud voice to the four angels, to whom it was given to hurt the earth, and the sea, saying, "Hurt not the earth, neither the sea, nor the trees, till we have sealed the servants of our God in their foreheads." And I heard the number of them, which were sealed: *and there were* sealed a hundred, *and* forty, *and* four thousand of all the tribes of the children of Israel. Of the tribe of Judah *were* sealed twelve thousand. Of the tribe of Reuben *were* sealed twelve thousand. Of the tribe of Gad *were* sealed twelve thousand. Of the tribe of Asher *were* sealed twelve thousand. Of the tribe of Naphtali *were* sealed twelve thousand. Of the tribe of Manasseh *were* sealed twelve thousand. Of the tribe of Simeon *were* sealed twelve thousand.

Of the tribe of Levi *were* sealed twelve thousand. Of the tribe of Issachar *were* sealed twelve thousand. Of the tribe of Zebulun *were* sealed twelve thousand. Of the tribe of Joseph *were* sealed twelve thousand. Of the tribe of Benjamin *were* sealed twelve thousand. After this I beheld, and, lo, a great multitude, which no man could number, of all nations, and kindreds, and people, and tongues, stood before the throne, and before the Lamb, clothed with white robes, and palms in their hands; and cried with a loud voice, saying, Salvation to our God, which sitteth upon the throne, and unto the Lamb. And all the angels stood round about the throne, and *about* the elders, and the four beasts, and fell before the throne on their faces, and worshipped God, saying, Amen: Blessing, and glory, and wisdom, and thanksgiving, and honour, and power, and might, *be* unto our God for ever and ever. Amen. And one of the elders answered, saying unto me, "What are these, which are arrayed in white robes? And whence came they?" And I said unto him, "Sir, thou knowest." And he said to me, "These are they, which came out of great tribulation, and have washed their robes, and made them white in the blood of the Lamb. Therefore, are they before the throne of God, and serve him day, and night, in his temple: and he that sitteth on the throne shall dwell among them. They shall hunger no more, neither thirst anymore; neither shall the sun light on them, nor any heat.

For the Lamb, which is in the midst of the throne shall feed them, and shall lead them unto living fountains of waters: and God shall wipe away all tears from their eyes." And when he had opened the seventh seal, there was silence in heaven about the space of half an hour. And I saw the seven angels, which stood before God; and to them were given seven trumpets. And another angel came, and stood at the altar, having a golden censer; and there was given unto him much incense, that he should offer *it,* with the prayers of all saints, upon the golden altar, which was before the throne. And the smoke of the incense, *which came* with the prayers of the saints, ascended up before God, out of the angel's hand. And the angel took the censer, and filled it with fire of the altar, and cast *it* into the earth: and there were voices, and thunderings, and lightnings, and an earthquake.

And the seven angels, which had the seven trumpets, prepared themselves to sound. The first angel sounded, and there followed hail, and fire mingled with blood, and they were cast upon the earth: and the third part of trees was burnt up in nuclear war, and all green grass was burnt up. And the second angel sounded, and as it were a great mountain burning with fire was cast into the sea: and the third part of the sea became blood; and the third part of the creatures, which were in the sea, and had life, died; and the third part of the ships were destroyed. And the third angel sounded, and there fell a great star from heaven, burning as it were a lamp, and it fell upon the third part of the rivers, and upon the fountains of waters; and the name of the star is called Wormwood: 'Global Warming,' and the third part of the waters became wormwood; 'the polar cap melting,' and many men died of the waters, because they were made bitter. And the fourth angel sounded, and the third part of the sun was smitten, and the third part of the moon, and the third part of the stars; so as the third part of them was darkened, and the day shone not for a third part of it, and the night likewise from the dust of all the nuclear weapons used by the Politicians to bring to pass their policies of an one world empire. And I beheld, and heard an angel flying through the midst of heaven, saying with a loud voice, Woe, woe, woe, to the inhabitancy of the earth by reason of the other voices of the trumpet of the three angels, which are yet to sound! And the fifth angel sounded, and I saw a star fall from heaven, unto the earth: and to him was given the key of the bottomless pit. And he opened the bottomless pit; and there arose a smoke out of the pit, as the smoke of a great furnace; and the sun, and the air were darkened by reason of the smoke of the pit. And there came out of the smoke locusts upon the earth: and unto them was given power, as the scorpions of the earth have power. And it was commanded them that they should not hurt the grass of the earth, neither any green thing, neither any tree; but only those men, which have not the seal of God in their foreheads. And to them it was given that they should not kill them, but that they should be tormented five months: and their torment *was* as the torment of a scorpion, when he striketh a man, 'the diseases that man created by going in the wrong direction on the road to nowhere.' And in those days shall men seek death, and shall not find it; for nothing exists on the road going to nowhere but emptiness, and shall desire to die, and death shall flee from them. And the shapes of the locusts *were* like unto horses prepared unto battle; and on their heads *were* as it were crowns like gold, and their faces *were* as the faces of men. And they had hair as the hair of women, and their teeth were as *the teeth* of lions. And they had breastplates as it were breastplates of iron; and the sound of their wings *was* as the sound of chariots of many horses running to battle. And they had tails like unto scorpions, and there were stings in their tails: and their power *was* to hurt men, five months. And they had a king over them, *which is* the angel of the bottomless pit, whose name in the Hebrew tongue *is* Abaddon, but in the Greek tongue hath *his* name Apollyon.

One woe is past; *and,* behold, there come two woes more hereafter. And the sixth angel sounded, and I heard a voice from the four horns of the golden altar, which is before God, saying to the sixth angel, which had the trumpet, Loose the four angels, which are bound in the great river Euphrates. And the four angels were loosed, which were prepared for an hour, and a day, and a month, and a year, for to slay the third part of men. And the number of the army of the horsemen *were* two hundred thousand, thousand: and I heard the number of them. And thus I saw the horses in the vision, and them that sat on them, having breastplates of fire, and of jacinth, and brimstone: and the heads of the horses *were* as the heads of lions; and out of their mouths issued fire, and smoke, and brimstone. By these three was the third part of men killed, by the fire, nuclear weapons and by the smoke, their burning corpses, and by the brimstone, which issued out of their mouths.

For their power is in their mouth, and in their tails: for their tails *were* like unto serpents, and had heads, and with them they do hurt. And the rest of the men, which were not killed by these plagues, yet repented not of the works of their hands, that they should not worship devils, and idols of gold, and silver, and brass, and stone, and of wood; which neither can see, nor hear, nor walk: neither repented they of their murders, nor of their sorceries, nor of their fornication, nor of their thefts. And I saw another mighty angel come down from heaven, clothed with a cloud: and a rainbow *was* upon his head, and his face *was* as it were the sun, and his feet as pillars of fire: and he had in his hand a little book open: and he set his right foot upon the sea, and *his* left *foot* on the earth, and cried with a loud voice as *when* a lion roareth: and when he had cried, seven thunders uttered their voices. And when the seven thunders had uttered their voices, I was about to write: and I heard a voice from heaven saying unto me, "Seal up those things, which the seven thunders uttered, and write them not." And the angel, which I saw stand upon the sea and upon the earth lifted up his hand to heaven, and swore by him that lives for ever, and ever, who created heaven, and the things, that therein are, and the earth, and the things, that therein are, and the sea, and the things, which are therein, that there should be time no longer: but in the days of the voice of the seventh angel, when he shall begin to sound, the mystery of God should be finished, and that is, "look at your hearts," as he hath declared to his servants the prophets. And the voice, which I heard from heaven and had spoken unto me again, and said, "Go *and* take the little book, which is open in the hand of the angel, which standeth upon the sea, and upon the earth." And I went unto the angel, and said unto him, "Give me the little book." And he said unto me, "Take *it,* and eat it up; and it shall make thy belly bitter but it shall be in thy mouth sweet as honey."

And I took the little book out of the angel's hand, and ate it up; and it was in my mouth sweet as honey: and as soon as I had eaten it, my belly was bitter. And he said unto me, "Thou must prophesy again before many peoples, and nations, and tongues, and kings." And there was given me a reed like, unto a rod: and the angel stood, saying, "Rise, and measure the temple of God, and the altar, and them that worship therein.

But the court which is without the temple leave out, and measure it not; for it is given unto the Gentiles: and the holy city shall they tread under foot forty *and* two months. And I will give *power* unto my two witnesses, and they shall prophesy a thousand two hundred, *and* threescore days, clothed in sackcloth.

These are the two olive trees, and the two candlesticks standing before the God of the earth. And if any man will hurt them, fire proceedeth out of their mouth, and devoureth their enemies: and if any man will hurt them, he must in this manner be killed. These have power to shut heaven, that it rain not in the days of their prophecy: and have power over waters to turn them to blood, the wages of how many innocent lives were taken in war, and just plain madness, that man is God, and to smite the earth with all plagues as often as they will. And when they shall have finished their testimony, the beast, that ascendeth out of the bottomless pit, shall make war against them, and shall overcome them, and kill them. And their dead bodies *shall lie* in the street of the great city, which spiritually is called Sodom and Egypt, where also our Lord was crucified. And they of the people and kindred, and tongues, and nations shall see their dead bodies three days, and a half, and shall not suffer their dead bodies to be put in graves.

And they that dwell upon the earth shall rejoice over them, and make merry, and shall send gifts one to another; because these two prophets tormented them, that dwelt on the earth. And after three days, and a half the Spirit of life from God entered into them, and they stood upon their feet; and great fear fell upon them, which saw them. And they heard a great voice from heaven saying unto them, Come up hither. And they ascended up to heaven in a cloud; and their enemies beheld them. And the same hour was there a great earthquake, and the tenth part of the city fell and in the earthquake were slain of men seven thousand: and the remnant were affrighted, and gave glory to the God of heaven." The second woe is past; *and,* behold, the third woe cometh quickly. And the seventh angel sounded; and there were great voices in heaven, saying, "The kingdoms of this world are become *the kingdoms* of our Lord, and of his Christ; and he shall reign for ever and ever." And the four, and twenty elders, which sat before God on their seats, fell upon their faces, and worshipped God, saying, "We give thee thanks, O Lord God Almighty, which art, and was, and art to come; because thou hast taken to thee thy great power, and hast reigned. And the nations were angry, and thy wrath is come, and the time of the dead, that they should be judged, and that thou shouldest give reward unto thy servants the prophets, and to the saints, and them, that fear thy name, small and great; and shouldest destroy them which destroy the earth." And the temple of God was opened in heaven, and there was seen in his temple the ark of his testament: and there were lightings, and voices, and thundering, and an earthquake, and great hail. And there appeared a great wonder in heaven; a woman clothed with the sun and the moon under her feet, and upon her head a crown of twelve stars: and she being with child cried, travailing in birth, and pained to be delivered. And there appeared another wonder in heaven; and behold a great red dragon, having seven heads and ten horns, and seven crowns upon his heads. And his tail drew the third part of the stars of heaven, and did cast them to the earth: and the dragon stood before the woman, which was ready to be delivered, for to devour her child as soon as it was born. And she brought forth a man child, who was to rule all nations with a rod of iron: and her child was caught up unto God, and *to* his throne. And the woman fled into the wilderness, where she hath a place prepared of God, that they should feed her there a thousand two hundred *and* threescore days. And there was war in heaven: Michael and his angels fought against the dragon; 'Hell Boy,' and the dragon fought, and his angels, and prevailed not; neither was their place found any more in heaven, and the great dragon was cast out, that old serpent, called the Devil, and Satan, which deceiveth the whole world: he was cast out into the earth, and his angels were cast out with him.

And I heard a loud voice saying in heaven, "Now is come salvation, and strength, and the kingdom of our God, and the power of his Christ: for the accuser of our brethren is cast down, which accused them before our God day and night. And they overcame him by the blood of the Lamb and by the word of their testimony; and they loved not their lives unto the death. Therefore rejoice *ye* heavens, and ye that dwell in them. Woe to the inhabitancy of the earth, and of the sea! For the devil is come down unto you, having great wrath, because he knoweth that he hath but a short time. And when the dragon saw that he was cast unto the earth, he persecuted the woman, which brought forth the man *child*. And to the woman were given two wings of a great eagle, that she might fly into the wilderness, into her place, where she is nourished for a time, and times, and half a time, from the face of the serpent. And the serpent cast out of his mouth water as a flood after the woman, that he might cause her to be carried away of the flood. And the earth helped the woman; and the earth opened her mouth, and swallowed up the flood, which the dragon cast out of his mouth. And the dragon was wroth with the woman, and went to make war with the remnant of her seed, which keep the commandments of God, and have the testimony of Jesus Christ. And I stood upon the sand of the sea, and saw a beast rise up out of the sea, having seven heads, and ten horns, and upon his horns ten crowns, and upon his heads the name of blasphemy. And the beast, which I saw was like unto a leopard, and his feet were as *the feet* of a bear, and his mouth as the mouth of a lion: and the dragon gave him his power, and his seat, and great authority. And I saw one of his heads as it were wounded to death; and his deadly wound was healed: and all the world wondered after the beast. And they worshipped the dragon, which gave power unto the beast: and they worshipped the beast, saying, who *is* like unto the beast?

Who is able to make war with him? And there was given unto him a mouth speaking great things and blasphemies; and power was given unto him to continue forty *and* two months. And he opened his mouth in blasphemy against God, to blaspheme his name, and his tabernacle, and them that dwell in heaven. And it was given unto him to make war with the saints, and to overcome them: and power was given him over all kindreds, and tongues, and nations. And all that dwell upon the earth shall worship him, whose names are not written in the book of life of the Lamb slain from the foundation of the world. If any man have an ear, let him hear. He that leadeth into captivity shall go into captivity: he that killeth with the sword must be killed with the sword. Here is the patience and the faith of the saints. And I beheld another beast coming up out of the earth; and he had two horns like a lamb, and he spake as a dragon. And he exerciseth all the power of the first beast before him, and causeth the earth, and them, which dwell therein to worship the first beast, whose deadly wound was healed. And he doeth great wonders, so that he maketh fire come down from heaven on the earth in the sight of men, and deceiveth them that dwell on the earth, by *the means of* those miracles, which he had power to do in the sight of the beast; saying to them, that dwell on the earth, that they should make an image to the beast, which had the wound by a sword, and did live.

If I Am Then I Must Be

And he had power to give life unto the image of the beast, that the image of the beast should both speak, and cause that as many as would not worship the image of the beast, should be killed. And he causeth all, both small and great, rich, and poor, free, and bond, to receive a mark in their right hand, or in their foreheads: and that no man might buy or sell, save he that had the mark, or the name of the beast, or the number of his name. Here is wisdom.

Let him that hath understanding count the number of the beast: for it is the number of a man; and his number *is* Six hundred threescore *and* six. And I looked, and, lo, a Lamb stood on the mount Zion, and with him a hundred, and forty, *and* four thousand, having his Father's name written in their foreheads. And I heard a voice from heaven as the voice of many waters, and as the voice of a great thunder: and I heard the voice of harpers, harping with their harps: and they sung as it were a new song, before the throne, and before the four beasts, and the elders: and no man could learn that song but the hundred, *and* forty, *and* four thousand, which were redeemed from the earth. These are they, which were not defiled with women; for they are virgins.

These are they, which follow the Lamb whithersoever he goeth. These were redeemed from among men, *being* the first fruits unto God and to the Lamb. In addition, in their mouth was found no guile: for they are without fault, before the throne of God. And I saw another angel fly in the midst of heaven, having the everlasting gospel to preach unto them, that dwell on the earth, and to every nation, and kindred, and tongue, and people, saying with a loud voice, "Fear God, and give glory to him; for the hour of his judgment is come: and worship him, that made heaven, and earth, and the sea, and the fountains of waters." Moreover, there followed another angel, saying, "Babylon is fallen, is fallen, that great city, because she made all nations drink of the wine of the wrath of her fornication." And the third angel followed them, saying with a loud voice, "If any man worship the beast, and his image, the image of commerce, and receive *his* mark of commerce, without a conscience in his forehead, or in his hand, the same shall drink of the wine of the wrath of God, which is poured out without mixture into the cup of his indignation; and he shall be tormented with fire and brimstone, in the presence of the holy angels, and in the presence of the Lamb: and the smoke of their torment ascendeth up for ever and ever: and they have no rest day nor night, who worship the beast and his image, and whosoever receiveth the mark of his name." Here is the patience of the saints: here *are* they that keep the commandments of God, and the faith of Jesus. And I heard a voice from heaven saying unto me, Write, Blessed *are* the dead, which die in the Lord from henceforth: "Yea," saith the Spirit, "that they may rest from their labours; and their works do follow them." And I looked, and behold a white cloud, and upon the cloud *one* sat like unto the Son of man, having on his head a golden crown, and in his hand a sharp sickle. And another angel came out of the temple, crying with a loud voice to him that sat on the cloud, "Thrust in thy sickle, and reap: for the time is come for thee to reap; for the harvest of the earth is ripe." And he that sat on the cloud, thrust in his sickle, on the earth; and the earth was reaped. And another angel came out of the temple, which is in heaven, he also having a sharp sickle. And another angel came out from the altar, which had power over fire; and cried with a loud cry to him that had the sharp sickle, saying, "Thrust in thy sharp sickle, and gather the clusters of the vine of the earth; for her grapes are fully ripe."

And the angel thrust in his sickle into the earth, and gathered the vine of the earth, and cast *it* into the great winepress of the wrath of God. And the winepress was trodden without the city, and blood came out of the winepress, even unto the horse bridles, by the space of a thousand, *and* six hundred furlongs. And I saw another sign in heaven, great and marvellous, seven angels having the seven last plagues; for in them is filled up the wrath of God. And I saw as it were a sea of glass mingled with fire: and them that had gotten the victory over the beast, and over his image, and over his mark, *and* over the number of his name, stand on the sea of glass, having the harps of God. And they sang the song of Moses, the servant of God, and the song of the Lamb, saying, "Great and marvellous *are* thy works, Lord God Almighty; just and true *are* thy ways, thou King of saints.

Who shall not fear thee, O Lord, and glorify thy name? For *thou* only *art* holy: for all nations shall come, and worship before thee; for thy judgments are made manifest." And after that I looked, and, behold, the temple of the tabernacle of the testimony in heaven was opened: and the seven angels came out of the temple, having the seven plagues, clothed in pure and white linen, and having their breasts girded with golden girdles. And one of the four beasts gave unto the seven angels, seven golden vials full of the wrath of God, who liveth for ever and ever. And the temple was filled with smoke from the glory of God, and from his power; and no man was able to enter into the temple, till the seven plagues of the seven angels were fulfilled. And I heard a great voice out of the temple saying to the seven angels, Go your ways, and pour out the vials of the wrath of God upon the earth. And the first went, and poured out his vial upon the earth; and there fell a noisome and grievous sore upon the men, which had the mark of the beast, and *upon* them, which worshipped his image. And the second angel poured out his vial upon the sea; and it became as the blood of a dead *man:* and every living soul died in the sea. And the third angel poured out his vial upon the rivers, and fountains of waters; and they became blood. And I heard the angel of the waters say, "Thou art righteous, O Lord, which art, and was, and shalt be, because thou hast judged thus.

For they have shed the blood of saints and prophets, the poor, the innocent for a piece of dirt and oil and thou hast given them blood to drink; for they are worthy." And I heard another out of the altar say, "Even so, Lord God Almighty, true and righteous *are* thy judgments." And the fourth angel poured out his vial upon the sun; and power was given unto him to scorch men with fire. And men were scorched with great heat, and blasphemed the name of God, which hath power over these plagues: and they repented not to give him glory. And the fifth angel poured out his vial upon the seat of the beast; and his kingdom was full of darkness; and they gnawed their tongues for pain, and blasphemed the God of heaven, because of their pains, and their sores, and repented not of their deeds. And the sixth angel poured out his vial upon the great river Euphrates; and the water thereof was dried up, that the way of the kings of the east might be prepared.

And I saw three unclean spirits, like frogs *come* out of the mouth of the dragon, and out of the mouth of the beast, and out of the mouth of the false prophet. For they are the spirits of devils, working miracles, *which* go forth unto the kings of the earth, and of the whole world, to gather them to the battle of that great day of God

Almighty. Behold, I come as a thief. Blessed *is* he that watcheth, and keepeth his garments, lest he walk naked, and they see his shame. And he gathered them together into a place called in the Hebrew tongue Armageddon. And the seventh angel poured out his vial into the air; and there came a great voice out of the temple of heaven, from the throne, saying, "It is done." And there were voices, and thunders, and lightings; and there was a great earthquake, such as was not since men were upon the earth, so mighty an earthquake, *and* so great. And the great city was divided into three parts, and the cities of the nations fell: and great Babylon came in remembrance before God, to give unto her the cup of the wine of the fierceness of his wrath. And every island fled away, and the mountains were not found. And there fell upon men a great hail out of heaven, *every stone,* about the weight of a talent: and men blasphemed God, because of the plague of the hail; for the plague thereof was exceeding great. And there came one of the seven angels, which had the seven vials, and talked with me, saying unto me, "Come hither; I will show unto thee the judgment of the great whore that sitteth upon many waters; with whom the kings of the earth have committed fornication, and the inhabitants of the earth have been made drunk with the wine of her fornication."

So he carried me away in the spirit into the wilderness: and I saw a woman sit upon a scarlet-coloured beast, full of names of blasphemy, having seven heads and ten horns. And the woman was arrayed in purple, and scarlet colour, and decked with gold and precious stones and pearls, having a golden cup in her hand, full of abominations, and filthiness of her fornication: and upon her forehead *was* a name written, Mystery, Babylon the great, the mother of harlots, and abominations of the earth. And I saw the woman drunken with the blood of the saints, and with the blood of the martyrs of Jesus. And when I saw her, I wondered with great admiration. And the angel said unto me, "Wherefore didst thou marvel? I will tell thee the mystery of the woman, and of the beast that carrieth her, which hath the seven heads and ten horns. The beast that thou sawest was, and is not; and shall ascend out of the bottomless pit, and go into perdition: and they that dwell on the earth shall wonder, whose names were not written in the book of life from the foundation of the world, when they behold the beast, that was, and is not, and yet is. And here *is* the mind, which hath wisdom. The seven heads are seven mountains, on which the woman sitteth. And there are seven kings: five are fallen, and one is, *and* the other is not yet come; and when he cometh, he must continue a short space. And the beast, that was, and is not, even he is the eighth, and is of the seven, and goeth into perdition. And the ten horns, which thou sawest, are ten kings, which have received no kingdom as yet but receive power as kings, one hour with the beast. These have one mind, and shall give their power, and strength unto the beast.

These shall make war with the Lamb, and the Lamb shall overcome them: for he is Lord of lords, and King of kings: and they that are with him *are* called, and chosen, and faithful." And he saith unto me, "The waters, which thou sawest, where the whore sitteth, are peoples, and multitudes, and nations, and tongues. And the ten horns, which thou sawest upon the beast, these shall hate the whore, and shall make her desolate, and naked, and shall eat her flesh, and burn her with fire. For God hath put in their hearts to fulfil his will, and to agree, and give their kingdom unto the beast, until the words of God shall be fulfilled," "look at your hearts." "And the woman, which thou sawest is that great city, which reigneth over the kings of the earth." And after these things I saw another angel come down from heaven, having great power; and the earth was lightened with his glory. And he cried mightily with a strong voice, saying, "Babylon the great is fallen, is fallen, and is become the habitation of devils, and the hold of every foul spirit, and a cage of every unclean, and hateful bird.

For all nations have drunk of the wine of the wrath of her fornication, and the kings of the earth have committed fornication with her, and the merchants of the earth are waxed rich through the abundance of her delicacies." And I heard another voice from heaven, saying, "Come out of her, my people, that ye be not partakers of her sins, and that ye receive not of her plagues. For her sins have reached unto heaven, and God hath remembered her iniquities. Reward her even as she rewarded you, and double unto her double according to her works: in the cup, which she hath filled, fill to her double. How much she hath glorified herself, and lived deliciously, so much torment, and sorrow give her: for she saith in her heart, I sit a queen, and am no widow, and shall see no sorrow.

Therefore shall her plagues come in one day, death, and mourning, and famine; and she shall be utterly burned with fire: for strong *is* the Lord God who judgeth her." And the kings of the earth, who have committed fornication and lived deliciously with her, shall bewail her, and lament for her, when they shall see the smoke of her burning, standing afar off, for the fear of her torment, saying, "Alas, alas, that great city Babylon, that mighty city! For in one hour is thy judgment come." And the merchants of the earth shall weep, and mourn over her; for no man buyeth their merchandise anymore: the merchandise of gold, and silver, and precious stones, and of pearls, and fine linen, and purple, and silk, and scarlet, and all thyine wood, and all manner vessels of ivory, and all manner vessels of most precious wood, and of brass, and iron, and marble, and cinnamon, and odours, and ointments, and frankincense, and wine, and oil, and fine flour, and wheat, and beasts, and sheep, and horses, and chariots, and slaves, and souls of men. And the fruits, that thy soul lusted after are departed from thee, and all things, which were dainty, and goodly are departed from thee, and thou shalt find them no more at all. The merchants of these things, which were made rich by her, shall stand afar off for the fear of her torment, weeping, and wailing, and saying, Alas, alas, that great city, that was clothed in fine linen, and purple, and scarlet, and decked with gold, and precious stones, and pearls!

For in one hour so great riches is come to nought. And every shipmaster, and all the company in ships, and sailors, and as many as trade by sea, stood afar off, and cried when they saw the smoke of her burning, saying, "What *city is* like unto this great city!" And they cast dust on their heads, and cried, weeping and wailing, saying, "Alas, alas, that great city, wherein were made rich all that had ships in the sea by reason of her costliness! For in one hour is she made desolate." Rejoice over her, *thou* heaven, and *ye* holy apostles, and prophets; for God hath avenged you on her. And a mighty angel took up a stone like a great millstone, and cast *it* into the sea, saying, Thus with violence shall that great city Babylon be thrown down, and shall be found no more at all. And the voice of harpers, and musicians, and of pipers, and trumpeters, shall be heard no more at all in thee; and no craftsman, of whatsoever craft *he be,* shall be found anymore in thee; and the sound of a millstone shall be heard no more at all in thee; and the light of a candle shall shine no more at all in thee; and the voice of the bridegroom, and of the bride shall be heard no more at all in thee: for thy merchants were the great men of the earth; for by thy sorceries were all nations deceived. And in her was found the blood of prophets, and of saints, and of all that were slain upon the earth. And after these things I heard a great voice of much people in heaven, saying, Alleluia; Salvation, and glory, and honour, and power, unto the Lord our God: for true and righteous *are* his judgments; for he hath judged the great whore, which did corrupt the earth with her fornication, and hath avenged the blood of his servants at her hand. And again they said, Alleluia.

And her smoke rose up for ever and ever. And the four, and twenty elders, and the four beasts fell down, and worshipped God, that sat on the throne, saying, Amen; Alleluia. And a voice came out of the throne, saying, Praise our God, all ye his servants, and ye that fear him, both small, and great. And I heard as it were the voice of a great multitude, and as the voice of many waters, and as the voice of mighty thundering, saying, "Alleluia: for the Lord God omnipotent reigneth. Let us be glad and rejoice, and give honour to him: for the marriage of the Lamb has come, and his wife hath made herself ready." And to her was granted, that she should be arrayed in fine linen, clean, and white: for the fine linen is the righteousness of saints. And he saith unto me, "Write, Blessed *are* they, which are called unto the marriage supper of the Lamb." And he saith unto me, "These are the true sayings of God." And I fell at his feet to worship him. And he said unto me, "See *thou do it* not: I am thy fellow servant, and of thy brethren that have the testimony of Jesus: worship God: for the testimony of Jesus is the spirit of prophecy.""

Chapter 23

And as I wait for this climatic event to happen, I compose my epitaph to go on my tomb stone as a memorial to those who got nothing from this life but endless regret, high taxes, woes, and great sorrows. The homeless, the wino, and the poor farmer whose land is stolen from him, to make commerce, and so he has nothing to make a living, to feed his family. The poor widow who's husband is killed in a bomb explosion, while trying to make an honest day's living, to feed his family. The neglected child who has to wash, and drink from dirty water, while those who are rich sit in front of their television sets, and watch in documentaries, the end of the poor, homeless, and generally those who are suffering. Kind of like a great big moving museum of colours and shapes and sounds.

Horace James Smith Epitaph, "Waiting for death"

You politicians, have you not prepared us well for hell?

I wake in the morning, and smell hell on my breath, and my unwashed flesh. Then, I am used to that. Then I can bear the smell of my rotting flesh in hell, as it burns in the lake of fire.

I am tormented day and night for all my years of my life, by my enemies, that is your policies of economic progression, that is, 'I must loose my home, where I raised my family as an honest hard working member of this country, because you politicians did not do your jobs, with the banks, and so you rather side with greed as they take my home for a piece of paper, which tells us what you politicians really think of us as flesh, and blood as to a piece of paper, that pays your salaries, when you leave office to go into the private sector.' Now it never ceases, would my torment cease in hell? Is there a distinction between night, and day there? Then you have prepared me well, you politicians.

I cry in the night, and in the day, and my heart is bruised, wounded unto death. Then my tears will quench my thirst in hell. I thank you all you politicians for that one mercy.

I am alone in my lonely walk upon the earth, and no one cares. Will anyone care for me in hell? Then you have done your job well politicians. Just as you said let there be light of your credit system, that now sucks my life, and my family dry, and you saw, that it was good, nothing wanting, then my descent into hell is so. For you never change, it is perfect. Have I not shown you your great and mighty wisdom here?

Politicians in my shame that you have placed upon me. I have been denied the pleasure of this life so that I will be content in the flames of the fires of hell. Am I not ripe for plucking?

Politicians, what more must I suffer, before I enter into the region of the dam? I sing songs of great sorrow, and endless regret, of pain, and emptiness all the days of my life, the shame that I have to bear for my sins. Therefore, you have provided me with entertainment for my sentence, in this great mighty prison, that you have prepared for me.

Poem of Repentance

Father, one door that you can close is the door that you may or may not have opened for me at Kensington Temple, for their past dealings with others and those like me. The truth is I rather burn in hell, than be apart or be associated with this kind of church. Why should my rights to Christ be destroyed there, and my life be in vain for them? The fact is my heritage in Christ is destroyed; there is nothing for me to gain by living for Christ. What good are they to you? Do they obey your word? Do they seek your face? Do they even know who they are in Christ? They let Satan rule over them for a lack of knowledge, and the question is, are they trying to change? They are a curse to what I believe, and me. They stand thinking that they are in your presence with favour, abounding, is this so? Then why is my life vain for them? One thing they have taught me is not to care whether I have favour with you, because I know if my race is in vain, and then I will burn in hell as I have given my word to my enemies, and that same word was given to you. Therefore, it stills stands, and cannot be changed. However, only you know whether I have lived in vain as I have believe, it might be said, yes I would like to spend eternity in heave but I have sworn I will not go there being defeated by your church, and how they allow my enemies to rule over them, thus destroying your providence in my life at the age of 10. I will stand in shame in hell, for this vain life, this is my word it was given many days ago, and cannot be changed, since I do not have favour with you. I will not ask you for mercy. What would be the point? Did you not say you will bless those whom you please? To your servant Moses. Then what am I in your presence but a curse. If that is not true, then why did Jesus have to die for my sins? Don't you think it hurts to know that as I stand in your presence, that my life is in vain for what is it, you cannot acknowledge my sufferings, my hurts, my disgrace, because I do not exist in your mind. It is Christ that you see.

Therefore, I am cursed to live in vain. Did you not say that your friends you speak to face-to-face? Concerning Moses. Do you speak to me face to face? Or are your words to me a mere dark speech? Confusion that you create in me for your displeasure, because if you were truly please, I would stand in the light as Moses, Daniel or even Abraham. Therefore, I must mourn, and declare a fast of sorrow, and tears, because of your shame towards me. If it were not so, then why are you silent, when I cry onto you my Lord? Why is my life in vain? Why am I alone? David your servant, after your own heart, did you not comfort him by giving him an army of friends, wives? Am I lest than a servant? Am I a dog? If he was a servant, and I am a son, then why are you ashamed of me? Why is your ways confusion before me? Than what is my life worth to you, even the excrement that comes out of the ass of your children has a better place to rest; it is treated with respect, more so than I.

When a dog is lost does not its master put out notices to find it? Does not he put out a reward? Do not they send out a search party to find that one dog? When I was lost to you whom did you send? What was the reward? Now do you understand why I say, that I am just a vain memory in your sight? I have to come to your presence, ashamed of what I have become. Yes the blood of your son can cleanse my spirit, and conscience, but it can never erase the pain of the shame, that I have become in your eyes. Yes it is no more but I have a memory Father, which leads to my heart, which leads to my conscience, and my memory remembers what I am. It can never change, not ever; this is the curse that I refer to you about. The sad fact is there is nothing you can do but give the order to your powerful holy angels to cast me into the furnace that burns with fire, and brimstone. I mean what am I to them? They saw what I did, they remember yes Father you cannot hide this from me, and what is really on your powerful angel Michael's mind? This is it, "it is he, (me), who murdered my Lord, therefore, and when he falls I will slay him."

He remembers what I did, and I will not forget. If that was not so then why did Paul write, that angels want to look into our salvation, because they don't understand it. They remember his death, and they know who caused it, me. Then who is their loyalty to? Me or Jesus? If I say slay Jesus would they obey? If Jesus tells Michael to slay me will he argue my case before Jesus? Would he intercede for me and why? What am I in your presence but filth? Did I not kill their Lord, and King? Then who is their love and loyalty to? It is Jesus. And remember this Father, if their loyalty is to Jesus, then where does your heart lay, is it not with your son too? Then I ask you again for I already know, what am I in your presence but a filthy rag, a stain on the conscience of heaven, for was not earth, and heavens created through His mind? Then what do the heavens, the stars, the earth, rain, sun really think of me? They hate me. They know that I am just a vain insult in their presence. If it was not so, then if I stay out in the sun too long, will I not burn to death through cancer? Yes Satan has a part to do with it.

If I go to the North Pole, will I not freeze to death? If I walk into the sea, will I not drown? If I jump off a mountain, will I not die in a horrible death? Then I ask you what good am I to you, because you see not nor do you acknowledge me. You say, that the world was created for me in Psalm 8, but if it rises up in anger, against my sins against a holy God, which was to slay the innocent Christ, would I not die in a horrible, and terrible death? Then what am I really to you Father? What am I, I have no favour in this world, to your church. And does your church ever see me? No, instead they retreat into the country. They neither see me nor know me, then I ask you what I am in your presence but shamed. Then Father why won't you let me die, and disappear into the void of nothing, where my torment can begin. Where I know what I suspect, now that there is no hope for one such as me. If so where am I to go Father? For 32 years it has been the same just a vain memory in the corridors of time. I cannot undo the murder I committed two thousand years ago, then why do I still suffer for it. For two thousand years I have suffered this shame. Now do you understand why it is easier to make the decision to burn in hell for eternity? Because I know now, I am made a prisoner of my conscience. I have no favour with man nor with you Father, it is time to die. Why do you make it so difficult, because why should I come to heaven, when I know what the angels really think? Are they not ready to punish any disobedience? Are they not greater than I? Then what chance do I really have? The truth is none. But a fading memory waiting to end for there is no hope for me. For I know what I really am in your presence? And what you have done through your great ministers you can do with anyone.

The truth is you really don't need me, and that is the truth, because you prove to me every day of my life. I know you don't need me. Every sorrow that comes my way, every hurt, that I suffer, every affliction I accept, every shame I have to bear, not from Satan's children, but from your church proves to me, that you do not need me. The question is why do you keep me, and not give the angels, the holy angels their greatest wish, to slay me in revenge for killing their Lord Jesus. Why not fulfill their wish. They want blood for the shame I have brought to your son, to mock me in front of my enemies, angels and demons alike. Why so you hold back their anger from me. Do they obey you when I cry unto to you? Do they come to deliver me from my affliction? Do they warn me of danger? Is it not in dark speeches that they speak? Is not in confusion that I hear? Then why do you torment me with silence Father? Is your anger at me that great? Am I not a mere mortal? Why is Satan, your enemy allowed into your presence, and I am denied it? Why do you tell Satan what you think about me, that I never hear from you? Do you dispute this Father? Then answer me this does, not your word says that you are God, and that you change not? Did you not tell Satan about Job without his knowledge? Then this is my evidence Father. Yes Satan accuses me falsely. Then why do you prolong my anticipation of your holy angel's vengeance upon me? Why do you wait Father?

I cry night, I cry day, but you are silent, in the night I am tormented by the darkness of your words, because I have not found favour in

If I Am Then I Must Be

the day. I am confused, because I cannot hear, because your do not speak to me in words I can understand. I believe I could accept my fate, which is hell, if I understood, why you have rejected me, in your sore displeasure, at least have pity on me, and tell me why I have been punished for 32 years of my life? Why is my life in vain, and most important, why must I experience hell? In this way my sentence is much more bearable, when I am cast into the lake of fire. I can tell the dammed, that you were merciful to me, and told me why I am cursed and dammed forever.

Father, did you take pity on my sins, and give me an education? Did you take pity on me, and give a companion through my sufferings? Then what good is life to me now? What good is your goodness to me now? Don't you understand I am but a vain memory to time, and that time is running out, and I draw more close to my descent into hell. Father can't you hear death, and hell calling me to come. It is almost time, they say. Then why are you silent? Yes it was my choice but what choice did I have. Was I not afraid of death? Then how could I live? It is only now, that I have had a whole church pray concerning a wife, you hear me, and then you answer me in dark speech, which I neither know nor understand. I ask you to show the light, and you are silent. Why do you hate me so Father? I cannot repent anymore. If you want my flesh or if I knew you would accept it as a sacrifice, for my sins for killing your son, I would gladly give it, and walk among the people of the earth as a freak of nature but you do not accept sacrifices, only obedience but if you are silent to me, how do I know, that I am being obedient? Why do you prepare my descent into hell Father? Did not Jesus die in my place to spear me from it? Then why must I go there? You allow fools and devils to stand in your pulpit, and I must listen to them, knowing, that I will burn in hell, while they live in paradise. They speak not the truth but in their understanding, which is dark. But you think you know, (Jeremiah 29:11). But to you Father I have confessed it to you, and if I go not you will be ashamed to call me your son. Would you not say I was disobedient to your word, because you said you gave faith to me, to believe you, and also to honour my words. Then when the fools and devils stand in your pulpits, deceiving me, who will save me from my enemies, when you are silent? Then answer me what hope do I have with you, and your church?

131

Father you say no it is not so then answer this question. Your word says faith is an act. Then why do you act to give me a pound to feed the poor, and myself but you give your ministers, and your unfaithful church, who deny me a place in your kingdom, good jobs, homes, partners, good cars, honour, and anointing that they abuse? Then what is my sin? Then what good is life to me now? My best years gone, and they will never return, yes you could do what you did with Job. And I know, that I am cursed, because I do not have that kind of favour, I look around in your church, and I see nothing then why do you torment me Father? Is it my blood you want I would gladly give it Father. But you are silent towards me, nor do you speak to me as a son but as a dog without a master. You never encourage me, nor do you change your anger towards me so I suffer in silence, because there is none greater than you, and you are just in the torment, punishment, that you have cursed me with. I cannot argue my case with you, because you are right. I am but filth in your presence. You made the earth, and heavens with your wisdom and you have put me to shame with, that same wisdom. And all my tears are just but a vain memory in your sight, because they cannot change you, because you are right in punishing me for 32 years of disobedience to your word. What chance, have I against a holy God? What hope do I have that you will be merciful to me, and have pity on me? The question is why would you?

Father there is so much pain in me that I care not for my life anymore; it is only the guilty conscience that I arise every morning hoping for mercy knowing in my heart that it will never come. Therefore, I just wait for the end of my life, when I am cast into the lake of fire, that is when your displeasure of me is full, and you release the angel of death against me. I just hope that it is soon, and I will know for sure that I am nothing in our presence but a dirty stain.

If I Am Then I Must Be

Chapter 24

He never gave up searching for what was lost in man, that became humanity, the love of God for all life even our enemies in him, that we would one day treat our enemies as ourselves, instead of trying to wipe them from the face of the earth in wars, famines, poverty, and diseases. As I gaze into the clouds, beyond the horizon, I see the ancient of days gazing back. But I cannot tell if he is smiling, because of all the glory, that surrounds him hiding him from our gaze, and beyond the clouds, I see the dark blue sky as gazing down, this I know is the Father's resolve to get his children home, those who have chosen to become man in Christ and not human beings in Saturn.

As I look at the trees in the crisp sunrays of God's righteousness. I see how the blacks in contrast to the light of heaven, that is now flooding our hearts, and minds, and as I look at the trees in the crisp cool light of God's righteousness. I see how black in contrast to the light of heaven, that is now flooding our hearts, and minds, and as I look at the tree trunk of the tree in the glorious lights of heaven I can see a richness in its dark opaque colours of browns, and blacks, and then the green leaves as they stand to attention, and waves to us as the wind of change begin to blow. But the very strong trees with large leaves on stand resolute only move slightly as the wind of change hammers them.

While the weaker, and smaller trees just move eagerly with the wind of change as change come to our once great nation that has now become the breeding ground of demons, devils, and fallen angels. We have become a ghost shadow of what we use to be. Like the 'City Mission,' who helped the poor. Instead, we see how the security forces help the homeless by moving them on to another place, just to remove the eyesores from our spiritual Sodom and Gomorrah city that we have created, just like the original one in the book of Genesis. And no one in the government appeals to our conscience for their sakes. And then all of a sudden the sun of righteousness breaks through in all his glory as right above me through the clouds the sunshine but only for a while and only a little about two feet, vertically from where I was sitting on the earth.

And what I see on the people the milky clouds is not who they really are, but it is the mist of the arts, and culture on them that is the power of the, 'Prince of The Air.' The entity that has blinded their minds to those who are perishing, because of the arts of culture. I can now see what the Lord is saying, that I am heading for greatness, because this is a very difficult realm to see in. I do not see it on my reflection of me in others.

Then I proceed, navigating my way through the army of traffic as I got to the stoplights after I had left Tesco I remembered in the evening as I was backtracking my way back to Tesco, two enormous blood red buses, clobbering each other as they honked their horns. Sounded the mating call, 'its clobbering time.' as I crossed over I get into formation as I listened to all the middle class students who wherein the subway shop, buying fancy sub sandwiches, because they thought, that this is what the upper class do, and because they were studying at college. They felt, that this was their right of passage, into the intellectual upper class of society. As they bought their 12 inches sub sandwiches, with extra cheese, and source on top. The price was beyond how much they could really afford but yet in their journey of fantasy they never ever graduated from the fairy story Jack and the Bean Stalk, which was my problem for a long time but I woke up just in time.

Then after buying my six inch sub sandwich, I head to my favorite spot, and that my chair of observation behind Nelson' Column, where I sit down, and watch the younglings as on this one occasion they tried to imitate the mighty great British roar of the four stoned statute of the lions of Judah, for a family photograph. Hence, they must be from a school in Europe that is fascinated with British Victorian culture. Then Nigel my very best friend comes over, and talks to me. He asks me what am I doing, and as usual, I say nothing. Just so that I can understand, and perceive what is going in his heart, because he is homeless. And when I think of what he has gone through I go back to my last night in Boston Massachusetts where I almost became homeless as I sat on my bed, waiting to end. As I get of the 159 bus at Trafalgar square, around the corner from Tesco, I head back towards the other side of the road first to Tesco to get my Coke Cola bottle, and maybe two Tesco trade mark cookies. And then it starts again for me the next day like, 'Ground

If I Am Then I Must Be

Hog Day,'

Chapter 25

As the instructor of thoughtlessness looks towards me, and beckons me on to answer his ideological question, on which race is superior, the white race or the black one. Just as one naïve white student mentions the word, 'nigger,' and an afro American male student begins to convulse as his deep down hate for white people, for what they did to him in his ancestors began to surface. This instructor of foolishness asked so bluntly, what do I think at this statement, that this white fool made, that being not sensitive to the past, which is still been lived in the ideological foundation of American culture today. First of all I told him, I did not come from the American black experience, I am the black European experience, and I cannot accurately answer your question, in the light of the ethos of the American experience.

This threw him, because the thought, that I was a black American, searching for an identity, when I had already found one, and that is the some of experience, that sums up who I am from the beginning when I first began, and it is not when I was first born into this world for Jehovah, through Christ said to Jeremiah,' "I knew you before you were born," I come from a further experience of existence, for I am now beginning to remember my God conscious, what I was in the throne room of God, before I came into the earth, to be one of the redeemed. When I left the, I am that I am to become what I am today to begin the journey back to that I am that I am. That is my journey back to the, 'Garden of Eden.' By traveling once again, the great distances of time, thought, and space in my Tardis, made up of the mental disease called schizophrenia. Where all is but a thought that trigger pain, hurt, emptiness or fun, joy, gayness of life, and or lust, sexual desire outside of the loving parameters of a godly union, defined in marriage to someone you love, not a part of your fairy tale life, and or fantasy.

I told him that I am European, and with European blacks, that were born there are outside of the American black cultural experience. Even though, in times of slavery, the European blacks suffered, just as much as the American blacks. But my parents are from Jamaica. My father has already departed this plain of existence, for another, whether to paradise, to spend an eternity with his builder Christ, or an eternity in the great and mighty prison, the lake of fire with his tormentor the, 'Princess of Darkness,' Saturn. I cannot tell. Then I continued on. I myself was born in Britain at St Thomas Hospital on the 19th October 1964. I was named Horace James by a nurse. Horace at that time meant victorious spirit, and light of the sun, and also keeper of time so I am a time lord of such. And James means wisdom, and supplanted.

My grandmother is African, and my grandfather is Indian, and I look like an Ethiopian. I told him, that I do not have the intuitive foundation as most black Americans to debate your request, for your quest for the perfect intellectual experience, that you will spend, the rest of your life, trying to emanate, while your fellow man lies in the gutter, dying or is already dead. But one thing I will explain to you, like an analogy. When you look into a mirror, in the morning, you see a reflection of yourself. You take soap, cream, shaving utensils, combs, and many more mind altering devices, to change what you see in the mirror, in the mornings, that you are ashamed to show the world. Then when you are confident with your appearance, you take it to the world as the real you, thus hiding the hidden you. In an illusion, that Hollywood, and advertising through the prophets of Baal, who's high priest is Jezebel, brainwashed, into believing, is the real you.

But in reality, is worship of a false God, a fallen angel called Lucifer. If you can understand, that all knowledge is parallel, then you will know, that this is true of when you look into another man's face, and call him a, 'nigger,' or a, 'yellow man,' or a, 'fundamental terrorist, sodomite, gay, murderer, women abuser.' You are looking at your own reflection of what you are deep down. So when the white Americans called the black Americans, 'nigger, and blacks,' it is a reflection of the white man's image of themselves, on the inside, that they are trying to cover up so when the Americans were denying the black Americans their civil rights, and lynching them for looking at their white women. It was a reflection of what the white race thought of themselves, on the inside, because you only can face what you have become in this life, and nothing else. If you have reached a place of peace, and serenity then you will reflect that what is in your perception of who you have become. If you only have reached a place of turmoil in your life, then you will also reflect that in your life. It is about changing the image that we have of our inner selves so that the outer image can change to one of love, peace, and unity for all humankind. Their African slave women as they were called then to bring their African black silk like skin to a nation that had never experience the African experience before. And so they turned them into slaves to breed for profit, while the black African man was broken, like a wild stallion, until he had no desire to resist the white tooth tiger's savage attacks, on his manhood, and fatherhood. In a sense what the black American man is now.

The white man made him so. So in a sense the black American man is reflections of the previous white man's deprave soul. And white men in America is a reflection of what the white stole from the black man, their spiritual identity, a sense of belonging to a mother land. In a sense, while I was in America, when I talked to the younger generation of Americans, they would always tell me, that they were either Italian Americans or Irish American Americans. But no one I met in the north side of America would want to accept responsibility as an American. Could it be that they or on an intuitive level, are a shame to admit, that they are Americans for all the blood they have shed, in wars.

Such as Korea, Vietnam, the cold war, Iraq and Afghan. The Spanish Civil War on the poor. Those who have no political voice in government, and the irony is, to be a white American, you have to identify with all the blood, that they have shed, to build the American dream, from other races, which is the ethos behind racism. And then the issues, and debate of the war of independence, and trying to break away from their parents, that is Britain. But as in a biological relation, we learn that a son is the image of his father so henceforth, America is the image of its father Britain. So in a sense spiritually there is not really an independence day until America understands that it is running away from a confrontation with America's true founding fathers, Britain to become like their fathers, and that is Britain. And then they come full circle. You cannot run from who you are to be whom you are. For all life, experiences precede from one point of reference the mind of God, in humanity, and not the human race, which is doom, by their own omission of guilt. But by coming to terms with what they hate in themselves, by what they project, on the world, they are coming to a place of healing of all nations, in one people, the seed of all nations, the United States of America. And most important, the war between black, and white, America in the movies in their lives, they always paint, in most cases, the British male the father figure as evil bent on destroying the world. But in reality it is America bent on saving the world that is destroying it, through wars and conflict, when the best way to bring peace is to feed the weak, build the towns. Not blow them up, and kill fifteen to get at three individuals, hence converting a whole village to the cause of hating, the west, and to destroying the American interest in the world.

But on the other hand, what would happened if we as the stronger nations, were to go into conflict areas, and feed the weak, the starving, giving them back, their freedom through love, and tuff love. Saying, "And you my son who I never had what would I give you. Firstly I would give you my wisdom in navigating the corridors of life from my mother's side of African descend and my father's side from the Indian culture that I love so much in you, and with your Indian hair, and your golden sunshine skin." And then my deep thoughts begins to overflow, about what I see at the pond at Clapham Common, as I, full of meaning, deliriously ponder the famous Psalm 23 in my distorted mind, that has been damaged by the products of humanism, a technique, that I learnt on my Access to Social Work at, 'Lambeth College,' again in Clapham in 2002. The course, that the idea of making oneself a better practitioner of the practice of Social Work, by looking a back on the day's or the week, or maybe even, if you are not too busy to ponder the day's events or really not too busy to ponder the week's events, then it would be the month's events, in a way, that promotes the classic quotation by that brilliant oration, of the apostle Paul, that we, as Christians, should not caused any offense to the Jews, fellow Christians, or even the gentiles.

As I sit by the pond, and gaze into the realm of the ripples of bliss upon the surface of the pond, as the sunrays refract of the surface of the tiny little waves as they wonder in the direction of the wind - blown by the course of God's providence. I think in my broken mind is this unity, and serenity, that I see at the pond, a reflection of who I am as I looked into the sun at the ducks, by the pond. I saw clarity even though the sun was very bright I saw a stance contrast of warm browns, and blacks mixed with the shinny metal objects, the cars as they lay in the sun getting a suntan without catching cancer. I guest the universe looks after it own creations. The sky was a pale with a giant British airways bird with a red tail screaming like an enormous eagle through the blue pale sky as it rides upon the wings of the Gods. And then as I looked out yonder, I see the white clouds going up as a vapor in a mist of pour brilliant whites, like in the tradition of the ethos of my spiritual ancestors the American Indians as they sent smoke signal to each other, and what where there whiter brilliant white mist saying as the sun rays came screaming down, with the heat of the flint stones, that makes the fires of tour, that burns so brightly in our eyes as humanism tries to extinguished it to creates a humanity devoid of the new man of understanding created in peace Christ's image in true man, a man of peace, and not war.

Not like the God of wrath, that the Israelites created in the Old Testament, that has frightened so many away from learning about a loving Father through the relationship, that Jesus had with his Father, and not the relationship, that the church has with the God, that they like the Israelites of old have created in their image. The ducks just skates along the pond as they meditate on their instructions from the great I am that I am, in the sunrays. The contrast of the strong blue crystal sea as it ripples as the winds of changes come to my life, for I no longer see in the darkness of humanism of the church, institutional learning, and politics, I see what it really is, and that is trying to resurrect the old man, that died on the cross at Calvary, with it old natures of jealousy, hate, racism, lust, and so much more, that was done away with in humanity, when Christ died for me, and those like me, and said to all who did not understand what they were doing, "Forgive them for they know not what they do."

However, I now stand in the light of my own reflection of which I am - now created to be. Then I notice a big brown, and brownish white duck standing just about 100 yards from me as he or was it a she cleans his or herself, and looks at the mechanical ducks as they roar past on tins. Their oceans, the highways of regression, back to their cave man mentality, and that is I Tarzan, and you Jane, and we are in the my home, the jungle of confusion, trying to figure out, what is a man, and woman, as they contemplate back, and forth, in their great decorum of their vogue like ethos, who's breast were bigger, who is the man that got laid last night in their debauchery world of lust sex, and drink, and of course drugs with a little rock, and roll, in their ocean, until they reach dry land, their homes, and their work places.

Chapter 26

And the trees they stand tall as in the day they were created, in the, 'Garden of Eden,' it seems that during the flood all life died except for Noah, and his family, and the animals in the Ark except I would think the water creatures, that could breath under water but the trees, and grass, and maybe even plant life remained. But now with humanism brain washing, the minds of the young to kill each other for glory, gory, and an idea that one race is better than the other, like how Charles Darwin came about with the theory of evolution, that one race was superior to any other race so all other races evolved from monkeys, who evolved from the earth, which is the core of racism.

But however, global warming, the increase in the world's temperatures caused in part by the greenhouse effect, and depletion of the ozone layer, just as the temperatures of the human race increases at the same rate into a hot steamy boiling melting pot. As anger becomes redder hot and explodes into a hot orgy of violence over the entire world. In protest, unrest, terrorism, wars, plagues, incurable diseases, such as HIV, that is the upper layer of the atmosphere from 15 to 50 km about 10 to 30 miles above the Earth's surface, where most atmospheric ozone collects, engrossing injurious ultraviolet radiation from the Sun.

Like the heart of the modern man who celebrates in orgies - drunken of reveries of booze, and sex while their fellowman is dying on the other side of the world, from starvation. Just as the change in the atmospheric zones from 10 to 30 miles above our heads, where we cannot see it humanity is dying out on the other side of the world, from the excesses of modernized civilization, that cannot be seen but in unfeeling reports from the news, and news documentaries as the famous words of the BBC, "We have to be impartial to the political situation in the Middle East as we report the news by not allowing the charities to use their broadcasting network to raise money for a dying people who have no voice in the modern world, because they are not considered wealth producing commodity." In the 1980s it was realized that mechanized pollutants such as CFCs the infantry of industrialization were violently attacking the ozone layer as the first wave of modernization of the comic forces of the universe as economic development begins to progress beyond the stars. But as with the ethos of industrialization the holes had appeared in the great experience of humanism, and the scientific expression of humanity that we evolved from a belief in a human based morality, a system of thought, that is based on the values, characteristics, and behaviour, that are believed to be best in human beings, rather than on any supernatural authority.

The concerns for people, a concern with the needs, wellbeing, and interests of people, the secular cultural, and intellectual movement of the Renaissance cultural movement, the secular, and intellectual movement of the Renaissance, that spread throughout Europe as a result of the rediscovery of the arts, and philosophy of the ancient Greeks, and Romans, especially over the Antarctic. If this is true, would not it make sense that our ancestor that is nature is now beginning to warm up things in global warming a little. To punish us for killing their other children from different races so that we in our racism, can be victorious, and then make statutes, and memorial to honour the poor who sacrifice their lives for the rich so that they would get drunk, and have orgies, and think up ways of taking all what the poor owns, like in things called mortgages, which is basic highway robbery, if you look at it, you are paying for the privilege of the interest on a piece of brick, which they will draft you into the army to go and fight some other poor fellows, for the sport, over a way of life called de - humanism, that is not freedom but death. Therefore, how far have our degrees of learning and of intellect taken us? That we would begin to believe the nursery rhymes, that we learnt as children as Jack, and the bean stalk, who some how sold, I think his mother's cow for some magical beans, that when planted grew up into a stairway to heaven, where he met a giant who wanted to eat him. Sought of like the fantasies, that you see on television of men and women marrying, because they have good paying jobs so that the wife can build her dream fairy tale dream, with her fairy tale babies going to Clapham Common to sit with their fairy tale friends to talk every one else' business but their own, while their honest husbands who really loves them are out hard at work, trying to make ends meet. Come home tired, and exhausted not knowing, that he is just trophy, like the man of the famous band with the Miss man who divorced him for a big payout.

Alternatively, how about Cinderella and her fairy tale white wedding, this kind of fantasy, I see a lot in America amongst the college, and high school students as they find out how much you are worth, on paper, before they get into bed with you, and if there are no appropriate specimens, they will find just what you call a dog to sleep with, to satisfy their sexual urges, which I can understand until the right specimen comes along, and then work all their charm to catch their, 'Prince Charming.' This was tried on me many times but my mother taught me well with her belt as she remembered how she was destroyed by whoring black men, who just thought of her as a piece of meat, and never loved her except for my father who did not even get a chance to marry her, because of the devil James Chambers who was an animal, and so put on his macho ways, which is to grunt, like an animal, because the woman is his, that is my mother, and so my father being passive left, and married the same kind of mucho woman, who used him to take care of her whoring son, and his wife, and their children.

As so not to go down the route, that my mother did not want me to go down simply, because, no one wants a poor boy, especially one with mental illness, I stuck with pornography. It was cheaper, and much safer than having a relationship that was not based on sincere love, and understanding for each other, despite our beginning, and sincerely working hard with each other's love, and support, and the support of our children, to build something from scratch, that we would be proud for our children to inherit. It would have been nice if it were a house, that the government did not take so much in inheritance taxes from, not because it is a just law but because there is no higher power to challenge their arrogance, that we human being, the poor, the afflicted, the miss – understood, are not just more than a meal ticket, to their egoistical dream of being Gods with a little power to make what laws they want, without the conscience to justify them in the eyes of man, and our true God. The God of Creationism, which is Jesus Christ, and their Gods of humanism, one of them, named Charles Darwin, and they say that I am mad.

What I thought Paul was saying to the church is that our enemies might attack us but when they do, it will lead to our salvation, and their destruction. Which does not quite make any sense? It is like saying that the whole non-Christian world is against us. Which as I learnt from my psychiatrist is one of the main symptoms of the disease schizophrenia which is my Tardis, that I travel the time dimensions of thought, mass and space with, and that is thinking that every one is against you. Which is what the church here in London, based on my observations as a leper, an outcast of the church as I have found out as I walk among the churches as a kind of Henry just before the battle that prove the English lion heart as Henry pretending to be one of his men, and he listened to what his men would not say to him to his face as so well put in the play 'Henry V' by Shakespeare, just like what the organized church will not say to the world to their face but boast of behind their backs but they voice their concerns about their fears in private. Then on that famous day, he gave his famous speech that encouraged his troops to fight with the heart of the lion of the tribe of Judah, with tremendous results. Nevertheless, in my case I saw how much the churches were hypocrites, when it came to the mentally ill.

How they would, at one church warn their members not to go to the mental health practitioners, because they only deal with mad people. And how at one famous church in Notting Hill Gate, a mentally ill young black man was ridiculed out of the church, and laughed at as he left very angrily as the second in charge of the church, who called himself a pastor began to make negative comments about his mental state, stating 'well he had a demon,' and so on. Then on that Sunday, he is preaching about the good Samarian who helped the stranger who fell amongst robbers, and thieves in the parable, that Jesus spoke of in the gospel, not knowing, that he was one of the travelers that held up their nose at the wounded man, and would not show any compassion on him. However, in the gospels Jesus said, that you must pray for your enemies, that God will bless them, because God wants them saved. However, God brings vengeance not us, and the things that I am thinking towards you maybe confusing but they are not. It is Saturn's religious men's, last attempt to stop the work of God going any further, and that is not the work of separatism or division as the western church portrays a relationship with the Father but the gospel of reconciliation for all humanity, no matter what background you are from but it has failed, because I am coming to a point where I do not care about worldly things. I care more about heavenly things as portrayed in all life, including humanity, animals, nature, and life in general. I have been doing some soul searching, and I have seen where I have made the mistakes, that have caused God not to honour his promises in my life. Now I am about to correct them. I saw and felt the felt tip wind of the cool breeze, in the lazy sunshine, of the cold brisk morning, in the autumn morning sunshine, at the window from the morning's daylight, the window in my aunt's house in America, with the wire mesh. The sun came in with a blinding gush of pure ecstasy as I bathed in the golden yellow sunshine, by the window as I laid on my aunt's bed who was my step mother, because she did not have any children of her own. A slut bag dog who was caught having sexual union with a donkey, back in her home country of Jamaica, wanted to marry her but like the Romeo and Juliet scenario, my grandparents were against it, for good reasons too. I mean would you want to, 'breed,' for a man who had his penis up a donkey's backside.

I would think not, you probably would not even know what diseases he would be carrying around on the tip of his love pen, that he writes his DNA monocles, 'the lens of the eyes of the sperms, that is contaminated with the DNA of a donkey, the in correcting of the vision of one eye's focus on what kind of children this witchdoctor would have had, my aunt bring into this world.' Therefore, with his primitive mind controlling gimmicks he controlled my aunt's mind to let her believe, that she had cancer and that she would never marry, which both happened.

It is the darkest side of this kind of entertainment called hypnosis. The hypnotic suggestions laid dormant in an inactive state, developing slowly until triggered, which happened when she went back to Jamaica with us, that is me and my eldest brother now dead from a ruptured spleen from drinking four bottle of Vodka a week plus twelve cans of beer every week until he just could not hold it anymore, and he bled to death. As I was saying until it was time for them to surface thus taking her life. With me, it was my aunt's husband who now has left her. On the day of my aunt's funeral due to the guilt, that I was carrying for her, you see intuitionally, I thought that I had let her down as you may know most Jamaican one parent mothers, always single out one of their best behave children to be their nest egg, their old age pension, and so I was my mother's

If I Am Then I Must Be

favourite, because I was so well behave, and so she would not let me be a normal child always blaming me for what her other three children did, and of course I got the beating, and so I rebelled, it was the first time, that I had ever rebel, and so in most cases, if not all, my aunt, my step mother would take my mother's side, and so I had to fight both of them. I was not going to be anyone's whore, after I had been sodomized. I was willing to even die for my freedom, no one will ever make me a slave, willing or not willing, I know that I only lived my life once, and I will fight to live it my way, and not someone's else's way just out of guilt, and that is what I fight for each day, and if it means me, 'as I am being alone,' I am happy.

Nevertheless, Uncle George said as they came back from the funeral, "You will never have any friends," and so those words stuck with me for the rest of my life, until now of course, which I do not mind, because based on what I have seen of relationships, I do not trust many of them, because they are fake. Most relationships are based on, 'in my world,' a need to be the boss so that the weaker one can be the dominate force, thus living as a Cinderella, in their own little fantasy, and I was not going to live my life like that. The psychic link of the shadow does not necessarily has to be connected to demonology but more so to your fears, and so you create your fears from the shadow of what you perceive in the dark of your own reality of your own reflection, masked in the face of your own id, that you see reflected in so many faces, that you think you understand in your pride not in true humility.

They are your own faces of your own reflection mirrored in the mirror of self perception in others, hence your Frankenstein monster of your own alter ego of personified to create flight in the human psyche of the soulish regions in my reflection of my own perception, I see a beautiful face, and faces of nature I like, most of all, to look at animals more so than the faces of humans being, because these faces of fury animals are like the teddy bear, that I never had, growing up in an abusive environment, where the Black Jamaican community was my enemy, my older brother was my tormentor, and my mother was my slave driver, and my father was never around to instil order, and serenity from the chaos, and disorder, that he created by bringing into this world, in one moment of his lust. Therefore, I suffered in silence, until I became mad with grief from the strain of the pressure put on a teenager from the age of ten but the good thing was, and still is I gave my life to Christ, and through all that I went through I really never went over the edge as do some who were in, and are in my shoes do, even though I had one stain on my enhanced disclosure as I found out when I took an access to social work course at, 'Lambeth college.' I did not get into trouble with the police again, that was because I was on verge of leaving for, 'The Promised Land,' 'The Garden of Eden,' in America, which I never found but by getting into trouble with the Police in the seventies was a heart felt cry for help, that no one heard so as I entered, 'The Promised Land,' of 'The Garden of Eden,' in America I give-up seeking help by my actions, and suffered in silence.

It was while in 1984, while at a two year college in Denver Colorado, that I broke down, and cried in from of an art teacher who took pity on me, and tried to help me but as I found out he was a Vietnam veteran, and so his pity was not entirely sincere, and in truth it was his way of atoning for those who he saw die in Vietnam, and those who he killed in Vietnam as his inner voice of his conscience screamed out at him day, and night, "Murderer, murderer," and instead of him coming to the cross of Calvary, where the one person we all killed has forgiven us he thinks like many of us, that he can cope, and mend by helping me as one of the Supermen of Mount Olympus as we see with the leaders of the past, and the future. And so he caused me more harm than good by trying to make me into his penance of his alter ego as it screamed at his soul from his heart, "Make him good, and you will have begun to atone for your sins," when Christ forgave all our sins when he died so he drove me around in his car, after college, which ended at 2pm piling me with his guilt ridden speeches of how he did not also have a father growing up, how he saw some terrible things in Vietnam, and I could agree with him.

However, I was hurting, and to be burden down with his stories of woe and misadventure did not help my situation, because I still had my psychic link to the shadow of the Frankenstein monster, that I was creating in my id, my alter ego a combination of Shakespeare and Hitler. I could not say no to his morbid charming personalities, for there were many, and so I continued to develop this monster not

If I Am Then I Must Be

knowing what I was creating or what it would become eventually around 2006, I saw it for myself it was a paranoid schizophrenic with the hearing of voices, and the seeing of delusional episodes, that has shaped my life, and thinking from childhood but one good thing is that I broke free from the psychic link, between me, and my Jamaican cultural roots, and I was free to be who I wanted to be, and that was not another product of my upbringing from a cultural perspective. I was free to be British, and not Jamaican.

Chapter 27

Then while I was fighting the psychic links to my mind, out came a fly being trapped, which could not retreat back to it colony, hence it became like a dried up spider, a small one. The sun got very bright, as it died from, a lack of blood or life, not the voices, but the desire behind the voices. And that was that I enjoyed them and fantasying about black naked women with big tits, when in truth it was the voices constantly, and everyday, and every hour, and every minute saying, "Give me some sex, give me some sex," and so I would not violate the covenant of marriage, and sleep with a woman out of lust to appease my captors, one of the them was my ancestral spirit in the form of Nimrod, the great Babylon King who was a great hunter, and hated God so he married his mother, and became the founder of the religion of Mary, being the mother of God but instead give them a fantasy, and not the reality as I would inflict great harm to myself in my one room apartment back in Boston to tell them that I did not want to go down the same root my father went, and that was to sleep with the opposite sex without really loving them, and then dump his responsibilities, that was me, and his other son, that he conceived in Jamaica, and go and marry a heartless woman who used him the way he used my mother for his sexual kicks of a man is supposed to be like, the Hollywood kind of heroic kind of man. For in the realm of karma, 'what you sow you reap,' and he certainly did reap what he sowed.

In addition, as the wind touched my right-hand very strongly, when I thought, how did, that fantasy get into my mind but not my heart? Not my heart but my mind. In addition, that was of big asses having sex with big black studs with giant penises, more than the cross of Calvary, where I know, that what I have become in my own mind, and fantasy killed Jesus, on the cross. I am this, which Saturn has placed, in my mind. However, as the wind from window blew as I thought on this one thing, why did Christ come to save me, what good is there in me. I thought on however, when this law planted by God in the conscience of man for our own protection is violated, then love becomes lust, and lust turns into sexual desire, and sexual desire turns into boredom, and boredom turns into sexual perversion, and sexual perversion turns into obsession, and obsession turns into, 'if I cannot have you then no one can,' and then the end, which is a complete breakdown of all the laws of the conscience, that stops the moral decay of a society as we saw Europe so fast turned into a amoral decedent society during World War II, where sexual fantasies became sadistic murder as we saw in the death camps, the impetus your wedding day in the ceremony, that joined two people that love each other together for life. However, when this law planted by God, in the conscience of man for our own protection is violated, then love becomes lust, and lust turns into sexual desire, and sexual desire turns into boredom, and boredom turns into sexual perversion, and sexual perversion turns into obsession, and obsession turns into, 'if I cannot have you then no one can,' and then the end, which is a complete breakdown of all the laws of the conscience, that stops the moral decay of a society as we saw Europe so fast turned into a amoral decedent during World War II, where sexual fantasies, became sadistic murder as we saw in the death camps.

The impetus there is evil as an active force, released by psychopathic behaviour. The main example would be the influence of Streicher, who derived sexual gratification from the persecution, and torture of helpless people. It is now called in a free society, bondage sex and sadomasochism. There is no doubt, that thousands of similar characters were attracted to membership of the SS by similar prospects. However, it is equally certain, that they were a small minority among all those involved in the Holocaust. Page 89 Hitler and Nazi Germany by Stephen J. Lee ISBN 0-415-17988-2-9-780415-179881. However, I believe that Stephen J. Lee was wrong in his facts that, 'but it is equally certain, that they were a small minority among all those involved in the Holocaust.' Because there is another Holocaust, and that is one of child sodomy, by those who have repressed emotions mostly found in the cloth of the Catholic Church.

This is the part, that the satanic ritual sodomy act was trying to create a vile young man who would sexually abuse others in me, and the main reason why I would not socialized with anyone for most of my young years as a growing man. But before the incident of sodomy on my person I said sincerely, "Christ come into my heart," and he did, and my love affair with the risen Christ, that is my fellowship with him by faith, and not a service to a dead God of a piece of paper, that is considered more scared than a person's life, and liberty as we have seen with the church throughout the ages managed to keep me from all harm, and making so many terrible mistakes of conscience, where you do not come back from. Like Sunny Odum as in, "Oh dam you sunny, for what you tried to do to me by trying to turn my sunny days into dark wintry nights," a recovering schizophrenic, that is I of course, and not Sunny Oh Dam You. I met him in a Londis store, at the flats, in Lyham road in 2006. I thought he was just afraid, and was sincerely looking for the address of where he was meant to be going, and taking his test for the Police Force, which evidently, he failed, because he was not intelligent enough to pass it, and he had a Masters degree in Business studies.

Nevertheless, he was too proud to admit, that it was, because he did not understand the English language, that well as he was from Nigeria who married a British white women, and somehow magically got his permanent stay in the U.K. But in truth, like my mother, he was looking for an old age pension as he was about 60 years old, and still trying to be a man, by trying to be a hero, by deceptive means, and that he was trying to take advantaged of a sincere person, like me, to intercede on his behalf, which I did not mind doing. I helped him to find a job, in social care, which he lost, because he could not do the work. Wherefore, he lied to me, saying it was because of safety issues, and those safety issues, which in fact were based on the issues of driving his clients, hence young teenaged adult with learning difficulties, to the hospital, and to recreation pursuits, and not having the training in the safety principals, that we need to pursuit such activities, safely but I knew he was lying, because the DVD, which I gave him of The Passion of Christ, he said he gave to his sister, when in fact he hid it behind his Snoop DVD. He told me that he was a Christian, and that the read the bible so I gave him a bible, which in the two years, and a couple of months, that I was in his presence, he did not even pick up once, and read.

Then to my surprise, when I went around to his one bedroom flat, that he had bought from the council to prove, that he is man but yet cannot even afford his own television licence, and he had out on his

If I Am Then I Must Be

lounge table a XXX hard core pornography DVD, which I know he got from the market in Brixton, because I brought mines there too, when I was being pressured by voices to do so. Nevertheless, I told him the truth as I am telling all the readers of this book the truth that yes I did buy XXX hard core DVDs from Brixton market so that every one who reads this book will know, that I am no saint, it took many years of soul searching for the truth, before I could say, that I do not watch these kinds of immoral forms of fantasies, that both degrade men, and women to the level of animals anymore. However, with me as I told him it was a wound that I had suffered in battle from the act of sodomy on my person, at the age of ten, that I was feeding, and not a desire like him.

Nevertheless, because he was in the dark as he prance in the dark one bedroom, that he lived out his fantasies of being a real man, shouting at the top of his voice, on his global theatre of his life, "All other races are beast, they stinks, they are animals," while he smoked his cigarettes, and drank his beers to a point, where all you could smell on his shouting breath, was the stinking smell of beer, and smoke, and his trousers down to his bottom as his unzip his trousers, in his fantasy of male pole dancing as he sings to the, Pussy Cat Dolls his version of the rhythm of the night, "If you think your girl is a freak like me then blow me," when in truth all he was doing was showing to his on lookers, how revolving he really was, and what he really thought about himself, in the mirror of perception as he dance in the darkness of his own destruction as he created it in the darkness that is the dark matter of his own chaos. However, because he was in the dark, and was the dark he could not see the light of what I was telling him. In addition, that was to look at your own heart. Therefore, on Saturdays, he would watch his native African women dance on the stage of his fantasy on DVDs, that he purchased from the Brixton Supermarket, and expect me to accept what he practice as being holy, and righteous, which I knew it was not. However, I was not there to judge him, he was doing a fine job of that himself. Because there is a different between someone who wants to change, like me, and someone who wants to enjoy the benefits of being a true Christian, and not change like, "Oh dam you Sunny look at what your heart tried to do to me." And the fact is I could not understand how someone with a Masters degree could not see this, and why he never had a job in eight years, and that was, because his passport, on re-entry to the U.K., eight years ago was stamped wrongly, and so he could not legally work in the U.K. We found this out together as we sought wisdom of why he could not get a job and with the applications, I had to spell most of the difficult words for him, and I only have a high school diploma from my high school, in Boston when I graduated in 1982. Then after time he sits down, and discusses what my mother discussed with him about my good nature being used by evil, and corrupted people knowing, that she was talking about him, when he had told me what she had said, thus sealing his fate, because I had known for many months before, that fateful encounter what he was up too and how he hid the DVD, that I gave him of The Passion of Christ, and how he lied about being a Christian, and so I continue as Henry the V in my commoner's clothing to see, and show him his real heart, and then in March 2009 I sent him what I had composed as my Epitaph as the slain Elijah, that many witches had believed I was in a poem form, and my judgments for the churches as I saw what they really did, behind closed doors here in London in Ezekiel Judgments for the churches, and for confidential reasons to not violate the data protection act I have changed the names. But in my rashness I sent him, and those in question in the poetic from of my heart's wound from battle as it healed, and I was able to see in what little light I had, what they were doing in the dark, because one thing my heavenly Father has always taught me is, that first learn to see the light, in the darkness so that when you stand in the light, you can see the darkness, in the light. And so in the poetic version, that they could see my anger at what I who is denied a place in their churches, and in their hearts, because of my mental health problem, and that I was sodomized, a place so richly deserved, unless I am able to contribute to the wealth factors, in producing wealth for them, by giving my testimony of being a well person, after God had healed me, and so I would have my picture in their faith newsletter, to sell the grace of God, and on their television programs to sell the grace of God, which is free, and which I would do even myself.

Chapter 28

Elijah's Epitaph is my thoughts put into words at the harshness of my captivity, by my mental illness. Since I have a deep religious conviction, it only seems right that I should take out my anger, grief, regrets, and sorrows with God, in the form of Elijah his spiritual champion.

Elijah's Epitaph

For further understanding go to Wendy Alex of God's TV here in London and her prophecy of a lamb seen in London, that was slain, this is what happened, however, it is not why it happened. In addition, the slain lamb, that was dying was in fact Elijah, and not the church in England as many are led to believe but in my fantasy. However as the Lord told me it is your choice to believe whether this is from a true apostle and prophet or a false one. My job is only to give you understanding so that you can make up your own choice whether to serve the real Christ or the Antichrist as so many have done in England.

Elijah speaking with God and his Father as he lay dying.

"Can the word of God change what is in my heart, when it is created in righteousness? Then denied living waters for 32 years, from your throne? Can a man who died from thirst be revived by words alone? Does it not take power? Does it not take resurrection power to raise one from the dead? In addition, what would I think if I am raised from the dead? If I have tasted the rivers of life, which flows from heaven? How can I understand it? It would be a foreign thing to me. Must I not be dead for this resurrection life force to work its full work? Therefore, I cling to the cross of my shame, tormented by my enemies. 'Where are the living waters that you seek? Why has it run dry?' As they mock me, with vengeance, forever hoping for life. Again, Father, I ask you why do you mock me with vain words. You say they are not vain, then why do they never come to pass? When you said let there be light. Was there confusion? Did anything interfere with its obedience to the word? Then why do you mock me with vain words? You said that your words shall never pass away, even though the earth and the heavens will, after you are satisfied that, they have satisfied you. They need to show that you are wise in thought, word and deed. But answer me this, if your word is greater than what you have allowed to be then why was I not in California to be ordained into your ministry by your servant? What was the purpose of your word failing? But you have said that it cannot fail, and must accomplish what you have sent it to do. Then what did you send it to do? After all, I am not your friend therefore; you do not speak to me mouth to mouth. Instead, you sent your angels in glory and power to mock the one that is at fault with you, and that is, 'I killed your Son,' and chose a murderer as my deliverer. Yes, you are not deceived Father for you know me, for you created me, and not I myself. How you continue to mock one with vain promises, saying there is light when there is not, and it shines but can I see it? Can I touch the sun in my darkness would it not burn me to death? Then how can I touch the sun of your righteousness?

Can I reach out, and touch the air and capture it? If I tried, would it not move through my mortal being to mock me? Then how can I capture your Holy Spirit? Is he not the wind, and air of eternal life? Then why do you continue to mock me Father? Today you destroy my hope in hope, by not showing me the light as you have done for 32 years as I have told you. You have done a fine job in preparing me for hell, the region of the damned. Will not I have a vain hope of rescue when I am cast into the lake of fire? But deep down, knowing that rest will never come unto me from above. Is it not so? Do I not cling to the cross of vengeance? My enemies pierce my side with their words to mock me.

They bruise my back for I cannot defend myself there, they torment my mind day, and night, and there is no rest nor peace. And you watch. Am I not ready to be cast into the fires that torment me now? Then why do you wait Father? You said that you will not suffer the righteous to see hell. Then answer me this can your words move me? For I know what I have done, and that is murder. I took an innocent life to save mines, and then have I not lost mines in the region of the damned? Then why try to deceive me Father? Did you not give me a mind? Can it not reason against the darkness, that you now speak to me in? You said light let it be, and when the light has had enough of my vain ways, does it not warms up the temperature to an unbearable degree? Am I moved? Do I not put on my sunglasses to hide my shame, and to stop the light, which is the forerunner for your glory, to stop me from going blind in my darkness? You said let there be rain, and there was. Can it wash away my sorrows? Will it even listen to my vain words? Then why would you think I am moved by your words of pity? Why do you mock me? If the sun, and moon, stars the rain sea, and land of this world cannot change toward me, and give me peace, then what can you do? Don't they represent your word? Are they not your ambassadors to punish me for my crime? Then why do you say I am forgiven, when I am outside your Garden Eden, looking in, and what is the wall, that prevents me from entering into your Garden of Peace? Is it not my darkness? The memory of my shame? Then I ask you again, what good is your kingdom to me? If a child is adopted into a family, when he is fifteen, can that child adjust? If he knows, that his life has been in vain? Then why do you mock me Father?

Then why don't you have pity, and end it let me take my place among the damned. I will not hate you for it." The words I heard Elijah speak to the Father in June 1998. "A person who is not lifted up with evil in his heart." The Father's replies to Elijah as he lies dying from the fatal wound that the Father struck: "If you have not seen the cross, you have not repented or more rather, you have never seen the full work of repentance in you. What happens a lot is that many come into the narrow gate by other means. Sometimes by guilt of another person or because they were healed, which means their motives for serving me as God are not true but based on their experiences. With the cross, it is not so. When you see the cross, you are changed, because you see what your sins have done to a holy man. Your sins killed a righteous man who did nothing wrong. When you see this, you will say what must I do," (The wind of the Holy Spirit blew upon Elijah gently saying to him as he lies dying, John 12:24, the truth is, a kernel of wheat must be planted in the soil. Unless it dies it will be alone - a single seed. But its death will produce many new kernels - a plentiful harvest of new lives.) "Lord to be saved the words of my servant the apostle Paul. And that just does not mean salvation as in the form of being saved. But as Paul said, when Jesus arrested him, 'what must I do,' in the terms of service to the king." Then I heard Elijah begin to sing to his Father on the 9th March 1999, "A wounded heart am I."

"A broken man am I. Dead inside with pain that is too deep to reach, it is when I listened to the harmonies of the dead. Does it rise to the surface for I am dead. I have born more than anyone heart's can accept for Jesus on the cross. And I am dead destroyed. Can hope come again Father? When will I be whole again? Is there such a thing called, hope for such as me? Alone, have I been, alone will I stay. Then Father I ask you, why do you mock me with your silence, saying, that I must suffer to be obedient. Can a dead man live or even feel? If I am dead, can I obey when you call? Daytime I mourn, hiding my torment in daydreams, and at night I am not silent, for I walk the halls of time alone, weary from battle. When will I rest for I thirst for true righteousness? I cannot find it in your church, therefore, I must ask you, is it a thing of the past? To come no more, where is this thing called holiness? Why does it hide itself from me? Why is this Holy Man called Jesus? Why is he silent, oh great, and mighty God? Do you not hunger to walk among your people again? Or have you lost your desire to touch the heart of man with your holiness, once more? Then what is this thing called the spotless bride of Christ?"

Then I heard Elijah reasoning with himself on the 18th March 2000: 'It is deep down in my heart, that I can say he has done me no wrong for there is no wrong in him, only love, which is a strange concept, which I am ashamed to admit. To even bow too for I am not worthy of such a holy man's affections. Therefore, I must hide, in my guilt, and shame until I am destroyed in self-pity, and loathing for what I am truly. Not in a pure man's eyes, such as the Lord Jesus Christ but in my own eyes. This I cannot change for it has stained my guilty conscience. And even his precious blood cannot erase the memory of what I truly am. Yes, it is true, it is written that if any man be in Christ, he is a new creation, and old things are passed away, and all things are become new. But in who's eyes? Not mines, for I did as I am accused, a sinner, guilty of the highest of crimes, which is to murder an innocent man.' The wind blew of the Holy Spirit was blowing on that day in the spirit. Then I saw Elijah as he composed his epitaph for his tombstones as the holy angels began to weep entitled:

If I Am Then I Must Be

Waiting for death

Father, have you not prepared me well for hell? I wake in the morning, and smell hell on my breath, and my unwashed flesh. Then, I am used to that then I can bear the smell of my rotting flesh in hell as it burns in the lake of fire. I am tormented day and night for 34 years by my enemies. Now it never ceases, would my torment cease in hell? Is there a distinction between night, and day there? Then you have prepared me well Father. I cry in the night and in the day, and my heart is bruised, wounded unto death. Then my tears will quench my thirst in hell. I thank you Father for that one mercy. I am alone in my lonely walk upon the earth, and no one cares. Will anyone care for me in hell? Then you have done your job well Father. Just as you said let there be light, and you saw that it was good, nothing wanting then my descent into hell is so. For you never change, it is perfect. Have I not shown you your great and mighty wisdom here? Father in my shame that you have placed upon me, I have been denied the pleasure of this life so that I will be content in the flames of the fires of hell. Am I not ripe for plucking? Father, what more must I suffer, before I enter into the region of the damned? I sing songs of great sorrow, and endless regret, of pain, and emptiness all the days of my life, the shame that I have to bear for my sins. Therefore, you have provided me with entertainment for my sentence in this great mighty prison that you have prepared for me. He prayed this prayer on the 9th October 1998. This is a dream that the Lord gave me it is of Elijah as he lay dying. The woman who was upset is his mother that is Mary referred to the meeting with her and Rick Joyner she told him in his encounter with her why her son was dying. The only thing that Rick Joyner did not understand what she meant, and whom she was referring to. It is the book called I think The Torch and the Sword. I have not included the words that he said to his Father in heaven that caused Mary to weep. But if you believe this is true, and read the record of the conversation between Rick Joyner you will see why. Remember this is my fantasy.

The Dream

8th October 1998

I dreamt that I was having trouble singing Mount Zion, so someone began to help me. I was looking at a woman who was very upset. Then we heard another voice. So the person helping sing called them over, and we all began to sing who were all dressed in white, and I was lying down, (words ordained by a man.) Something left me at that point.

But before he died, he said these words to the Father and the Father's response was to send back to the earth the glory that when Smith Wigglesworth was about to die said would depart with him. I think the Lord spoke in part through Kenneth Copeland and Kenneth Hagin about it. You can thank Joyce Meyers, for that it is partly due to what she did for him as he lay dying, many years ago. These are his words below to the Father of all spirits.

Prayer for the dead

There is no one on the earth to defend us oh Lord, no one cares for us, not even your church, which you promised, would not fail us. But it has, for we are robbed of our innocence, corrupted by his wisdom. We did not ask to eat the apple of good and evil. We were force. We were forced to slay your son Jesus. We cannot come to you for we are guilty of the crime, that the accuser has accused us of. So we fear when your servants pray for us, because we see the answers. Our sons and daughters are rape, and murdered for sake of wealth, our mothers weep day and night for us, our fathers are bitter at the punishment you send us so they die of a broken heart, for it was in vain. We hoped for deliverance, and protection from you. But instead, because you are angry with us, for murdering your son Jesus, you punish us, for we are evil and wicked. We cannot come unto a Holy God. Your leader, the one with the white hair, like your son Jesus, does she smile at us? No, because we know, that you are angry with us. We know if we speak to you, we are rebuked. Did not your church say we could not be members, because of our mental illness? Then we now stand in the streets, cold and wet, fearful of your coming anger upon us, with no one to save us from your anger. Not even Jesus can help us. Is it not in His name the church is named in? Yet they curse us to our faces, and tell us to leave, that we are not wanted here. "I am into you," they say, and we asked you for a piece of bread, and water that is all. We did not ask for even our inheritance, because that is lost to us. But do you hear us? Do you see us? "The answer is get out of my church you curse, you faggot, you whore, you mentally ill person, you might put me to shame. Don't you know your kind are murderers. You freak out in the streets, and kill good people, who deserve eternal life, because they have money to support our church buildings. If you come to our Sunday school children, we know that you want to abuse them, because you are not acceptable in our sight."

Then where do we go? We have no home. So we lay on the streets as we have been created to do and piss on ourselves in front of your church as we drink ourselves to death to drown out the screams of your son on the cross as he screams, "Forgive them for they know not what they do," because we have shamed your son, and so you spend 300 to 400 hundred dollars to send your servant to speak to a man, who has traveled to the stars, and back. We know he can fill you with so much joy, when he speaks to you of the stars you created that glorify a humble and precious God. However, when we die, and are separated from the world, then you will have peace, because you will remember us no more. If you could please spare us a piece of bread and water, it won't cost you much to send one of your angels to give this to us, and please say it is from your son Jesus, for we love His name. Don't you see how our eyes light up when we hear His name and receive the crumbs that are not even fit for the dogs from your kingdom? We are happy, because we know that when we stand before Him, to receive our punishment, we can say thank you, for just that one piece of bread, that you gave us. It gave me so much joy, that while we burn in the flames of hell, we are kept a little warm, remembering how merciful you were, even though, you did not want us in your kingdom, because your church did not want us. Prayed 28/11/98

The second prayer he prayed as he laid dying from the wound his Father inflicted on him:

Prayer for the dead

"How can we come to you, when we are shamed of what we have become? We are whores, homosexuals, lesbians, thieves, murderers, and more. We are ashamed of ourselves. When people reviles us, we cannot go, even into your churches, because your ministers seek those who can feed their lusts for there evil desires. Then they curse us by calling us sinners, when we already know that we are dammed. Life has taught us that we have nothing so we beg you Father in the streets, when it is cold, where we die, begging for mercy. Give us a little bread and a little water so that our sufferings be soothe a little, before we die, and go into eternity of despair. We see our own seed killed through war, when the rich are safe, because they were strong enough to seek education. So they become presidents and even astronauts. Then you send your servants to meet them on planes to offer salvation. They refuse it; it cost you 300 to 400 hundred pounds to get your servant there so that they could say no, because they are comfortable with their lives. But when we ask you for mercy, and we beg you just a pound please, you are angry with us. Do you send your servant to feed us? All we want is a little bread and water. Please, and that our seed be protected, at least when we go to hell, because of the hardness of your church. We are soothed a little, that we know our seed made it. But no not even that, because your holy law says that, 'if I am a whore, my seed must be one too.' Then you say we are cold, is not that our hearts are dead from our shame of what Satan has made of us? When you promised that, it would not happen.

Did you not say that you will maintain the cause of the afflicted and the right of the poor? What is our right? To live in peace, because the Angel of the Lord declared to the shepherds, before your son came into the world, to die for our peace, and it is not so for us. For who is the first to die in war? Is it not us? The weak, the poor who have lived good lives, but did not hear the gospel, because your church was too weak to preach it. They were too busy gaining knowledge and understanding of how to preach Christ, while we are dying minute by minute, second by second. And where are your mighty angels, God of all spirits? Where are they? Why are they silent, when I am old woman who have reared what you gave me, a child to carry on your heritage Lord. And when I am old weak, I have only one husband, who was murdered after I was raped, violated by a violation of your most holy law, 'Let no man put asunder what God has joined together.' Then with fire, I felt the pain of my screams as I cried out for mercy as I died to be remembered no more. Is this my right as the afflicted? Is this my right as the poor? To die, because your church preaches, 'Do not be burdened with the cares of this world. Just enjoy the financial abundance of a good faith life.' While I who never slept with anyone else but the man you gave me. Who never taught my children to steal or lie. Even though, I did not know Christ, but yet they can repent, because they heard the gospel. But yet, because the spirit, that binds my government, which you established to protect me, that I could accept your son, for his goodness, must die in flames, knowing that everything, that I have lived for was in vain. My husband dead, killed for a piece of metal. Is metal more important than flesh and blood? My sons starved to death in war camps, because of a piece of metal. Then answer me this. What was this so-called blood of the Lamb shed for? In Jesus name, I pray. Prayed 29/11/98

These were the thoughts spoken into speech of Elijah as he lay dying from a broken heart. "I heard in my mind, more faith, more power, and more strength. A powerful reverence of power came over my spirit, while lying on the bed, after this bitter prayer to God my Father. It was the power of love. It was slow, and I had to open my mouth as it came into me. While traveling to Kensington Temple, I felt that reverence of power in my heart. I have a certain degree of peace in my heart therefore; I know that I have been heard." Dream given by God 29/11/98. I saw someone get up, and he began to speak on the behalf of the poor. He was powerful. Then I heard my name. Dream given. 30/11/98 I saw myself speaking to the poor, and sending the blood of Jesus to feed them. I was standing, and while the words came from my mouth, they went forth with power and authority, which is just faith. I saw a mighty river of life coming upon me. The fire of God burned on my head. 30/11/98 Answer given on the 30/11/98 "While listening to Phil Driscoll something happened. A great chain was broken, and I saw such reverence in the realm of the Spirit. I saw the heart of God as he cried from his depth for the poor. I saw the heavens open, and the glory of the presence of God falling upon the poor, and the afflicted. I saw in my heart. I saw it. Then I remembered the Holy God as it is proclaimed in the heavens. I saw my Lord again as I looked into the clouds. I saw his joy. I saw his peace. There is a greater depth of holiness that has come to the earth, greater than the angels. It is the angels that bring it but it is God who has come. It is a holiday. There is peace, (rest, be refreshed). While standing at the window, I saw it, it's the window. I saw it. It is Christmas again, the birth of Christ. And the Angel of the Lord has proclaimed it again to all men, "Fear not, peace to you from God." As it was now, it is again." Then Satan said to Elijah as he lay dying from the wound his Father inflicted upon him, "You make me sick Elijah, you have changed the whole universe." "A new day, a refreshing not like before, (remembered a dream from the Lord about this day.) Holiness is now walking the streets of the earth, and I cannot turn away from it." Then he died, and then I heard the angels proclaim from heaven, Revelation 12: 10-12, "Then I heard a loud voice shouting across the heavens," "It has happened at last- the salvation and power and kingdom of our God, and the authority of his Christ! For the Accuser has been thrown down to earth - the one who accused our brothers and sisters, before our God day and night. And Elijah defeated him, because of the blood of the Lamb, and because of his testimony. And he was not afraid to die. Rejoice, O heavens! And you, who live in the heavens, rejoice. But terror will come on the earth and the sea. For the Devil has come down to you in great anger, and he knows that he has little time."

Let me explain the mystery behind why Elijah told the Holy Spirit to let him die. You will find the answer in Revelations 12: 11, "And they overcame him by the blood of the Lamb, and by the word of their testimony; and they loved not their lives unto the death." Now what did Elijah says twice to the Holy Spirit? Found in 1st Kings 19:10, "And he said, I have been very jealous for the Lord God of hosts: for the children of Israel have forsaken thy covenant, thrown down thine altars, and slain thy prophets with the sword; and I even I only, am left; and they seek my life to take it away." Now this is the King James Version, his testimony to cast our Satan. Now go back to 1st Kings 19:3, "And when he saw that he arose, and went for his life, and came to Beer Sheba, which belonged to Judah, (hence, refers to the Lion of the tribe of Judah Christ came from the tribe of Judah so in a sense the torch was passed from Elijah to Christ,) and left his servant there. But he himself went a day's journey into the wilderness, and came and sat down under a juniper tree: and he requested for himself that he might die; and said, it is enough; now, O Lord take away my life; for I am no better than my fathers." Satan was cast out, it is kind of like a self judgment thing, hence if my enemies in this case Jezebel is in the right then let her slay me, and in this case, Elijah was found right so he was the victor, hence his wish was granted, and that is found in Revelation 12:1. Now if you re-read Revelation 12:11, you, if you are the true body of Christ, and not the Antichrist's body you will see that Elijah did what Revelation 12:11 says, hence that why the apostle John wrote the words, 'and they overcame him by the blood of the Lamb, and the word of their testimony, and the love not their life unto the death.' So when you hear teachers in the church saying, that Elijah was a coward, it is not the Spirit of God speaking, it is the Spirit of the Antichrist. Because Elijah did what Revelation 12:11 says, and the other prophet that did it was Jesus on the cross, hence why Jesus said before he went to the cross, "I see Satan, falling like lighting from heaven." Now you understand the mystery behind why Elijah said he wanted to die.

Second mystery to understand:

2nd Kings 2:12
"And it came to pass, as they still went on, and talked, that, behold, three appeared a chariot of fire, and horses of fire, and parted them both asunder: and Elijah went up by a whirlwind into heaven. And Elisha saw it, and he cried my father, my father, the chariot of Israel, and the horsemen thereof." The key to understanding why this is what Elisha called Elijah, and that is father, and he said it twice. Now go to when Jesus is dying on the cross, what did he say, Mark 15:34, "And at the ninth hour Jesus cried with a loud voice saying Eloi, Eloi, lama sabachthani? Which is being interpreted, My God, my God, why hast thou forsaken me? Some bystanders misunderstood, and thought he was calling the prophet Elijah." Now you understand why Superman is called Karl El and his father called Jor El it is a derivative of the first two letters of the name of Elijah. Or more to the point of Elohim, hence which is the number 666, which is the Mark of the Beast. Who Satan thought was God now go back to Isaiah 14 in which God begins mock his ignorance, and what did God says he would do to him, and that is that he will cast him down to the grave, hence that is what happened at the cross, and

Satan knows it. It is kind of a summary of why Superman is the Beast himself. Now why this is Elijah's Epitaph is because Satan wanted to deceive Elijah into building his church in Great Britain, and Elijah would not do it, and so Satan kept pushing, and pushing until Elijah died in battle. In other words, he broke the law of the Sacrifice as when Christ was on the cross, and God said in the old covenant, that no broken bones in the sacrifice, hence he broke Elijah's heart, hence the spiritual bone of God. And that is serious. Now remember this 99% of the Christian churches in Great Britain are in fact influenced by witchcraft.

Ezekiel Judgments are a collection of some of the things, that I saw the British church practiced behind closed doors. And remember it is just a small bit of what I have seen them do, for approximately eighteen years of being in this country, and living with schizophrenia. Names and places are changed according to the data protection act.

Ezekiel judgments of the churches 12th March 2009:

For it is written, that judgment starts at my house.
1st Peter 4:17, "For the time *is come* that judgment must begin at the house of God: and if *it* first *begin* at us, what shall the end *be* of them that obey not the gospel of God?" "But know this you blind and deaf people, that I am God who created the ears and the eyes, therefore can I not see and hear what is in your hearts as I discern the thoughts of your hearts? I will encourage you all to read Psalm 94 in the King James Bible and lament on your future."

Hebrews 4:12, "For the word of God *is* quick, and powerful, and sharper than any two-edged sword, piercing even to the dividing asunder of soul and spirit, and of the joints and marrow, and *is* a discerner of the thoughts and intents of the heart." "And did I not tell my servant Ezekiel about you, and what you would do in my house of prayer?"

The Call of Ezekiel, Ezekiel chapter 2:
"And he said unto me, "Son of man, stand upon thy feet, and I will speak unto thee." And the spirit entered into me when he spake unto me, and set me upon my feet, that I heard him that

spake unto me. And he said unto me, "Son of man, I send thee to the children of Israel, to a rebellious nation that hath rebelled against me they and their fathers have transgressed against me, *even* unto this very day. For *they are* impudent children and stiff hearted. I do send thee unto them; and thou shalt say unto them, Thus saith the Lord God. And they, whether they will hear, or whether they will forbear, (for they *are* a rebellious house,) yet shall know that there hath been a prophet among them. And thou, son of man, be not afraid of them, neither be afraid of their words, though briers and thorns *be* with thee, and thou dost dwell among scorpions: be not afraid of their words, nor be dismayed at their looks, though they *be* a rebellious house. And thou shalt speak my words unto them, whether they will hear, or whether they will forbear: for they *are* most rebellious. But thou, son of man, hear what I say unto thee; Be not thou rebellious like that rebellious house: open thy mouth, and eat that I give thee." And when I looked, behold, a hand *was* sent unto me; and, lo, a roll of a book *was* therein; and he spread it before me; and it *was* written within and without: and *there was* written therein lamentations, and mourning, and woe. Moreover, he said unto me, "Son of man, eat that thou findest; eat this roll, and go speak unto the house of Israel." So I opened my mouth, and he caused me to eat that roll. And he said unto me, "Son of man, cause thy belly to eat, and fill thy bowels with this roll that I give thee." Then did I eat *it;* and it was in my mouth as honey for sweetness. And he said unto me, "Son of man, go, get thee unto the house of Israel, and speak with my words unto them. For thou *art* not sent to a people of a strange speech and of a hard language, *but* to the house of Israel; not to many people of a strange speech and of a hard language, whose words thou canst not understand. Surely, had I sent thee to them, they would have hearkened unto thee. But the house of Israel will not hearken unto thee; for they will not hearken unto me: for all the house of Israel *are* impudent and hardhearted. Behold, I have made thy face strong against their faces, and thy forehead strong against their foreheads. As an adamant harder than flint have I made thy forehead: fear them not, neither be dismayed at their looks, though they *be* a rebellious house." Moreover, he said unto me, "Son of man, all my words that I shall speak unto thee receive in thine heart, and

hear with thine ears. And go, get thee to them of the captivity, unto the children of thy people, and speak unto them, and tell them, Thus saith the Lord God; whether they will hear, or whether they will forbear." Then the spirit took me up, and I heard behind me a voice of a great rushing, *saying,* **"Blessed** *be* **the glory of the Lord from his place."** *I heard* **also the noise of the wings of the living creatures that touched one another, and the noise of the wheels over against them, and a noise of a great rushing. So the spirit lifted me up, and took me away, and I went in bitterness, in the heat of my spirit; but the hand of the Lord was strong upon me. Then I came to them of the captivity at Tel-abib, that dwelt by the river of Chebar, and I sat where they sat, and remained there astonished among them seven days."** The scroll that Ezekiel was told to eat is found in Revelation 10:8-11, it is the mind of Christ as found in the book of Ezekiel to the children Balaam, both Jews and Gentiles as the angel told Ezekiel in Revelation 10:8-11, that is the apostle John, that it would taste sweet in your mouth but bitter in his stomach, you are experiencing that right now you slow at heart as he said many centuries ago, "God is not a man, that he should lie and not the son of man that he should repent, has he not said it will he not do it?" And he said, through the apostle Paul that he is not mock, what you sow you will reap. Galatians 6:3-8.

Numbers 23:19, "God *is* **not a man, that he should lie; neither the son of man, that he should repent: hath he said, and shall he not do** *it?* **Or hath he spoken, and shall he not make it good?"**

And remember my servant Ezekiel was born on the !9th October 1964. That is why I chose verse 19 as my sign that I am not a man that I should lie and that I am not son of man that I should repent. I am that I am and that is omnipresence as David learnt in Psalm 139. The rest can be found by going to www.chipmunkapublishing.co.uk and ordering all from Chipmunkapublishing the works by Horace Smith both E Books and paperbacks and remember, the whole set cost about fifty pounds I will get about five pounds in royalties but Chipmunkapublishing, a mental health charity who are the dead trying to save the dead as what Jesus told those at Kensington Temple that the dead are trying to save the dead, and you the living are making commerce of the dead and dying, will make at least fifty pounds to help the mentally ill, make a living by producing E Books so that they can get back into a normal way of life.

A Watchman to Israel:

"And it came to pass at the end of seven days, that the word of the Lord came unto me, saying, Son of man, I have made thee a watchman unto the house of Israel: therefore hear the word at my mouth, and give them warning from me. When I say unto the wicked, Thou shalt surely die; and thou givest him not warning, nor speakest to warn the wicked from his wicked way, to save his life; the same wicked *man* shall die in his iniquity; but his blood will I require at thine hand. Yet if thou warn the wicked and he turn not from his wickedness, nor from his wicked way, he shall die in his iniquity; but thou hast delivered thy soul. Again, When a righteous *man* doth turn from his righteousness, and commit iniquity, and I lay a stumbling block before him, he shall die: because thou hast not given him warning, he shall die in his sin, and his righteousness which he hath done shall not be remembered; but his blood will I require at thine hand. Nevertheless, if thou warn the righteous *man,* that the righteous sin not, and he doth not sin, he shall surely live, because he is warned; also thou hast delivered thy soul."

"Now I ask you a question all you false teachers of the doctrine of Balaam as you now call it theology." "Who are the watchmen over the house of Israel?" As found in Matthew chapter 25

25 The Parable of the Ten Virgins:

"Then shall the kingdom of heaven be likened unto ten virgins, which took their lamps, and went forth to meet the bridegroom. And five of them were wise, and five *were* foolish. They that *were* foolish took their lamps, and took no oil with them: but the wise took oil in their vessels with their lamps. While the bridegroom tarried, they all slumbered and slept. And at midnight, there was a cry made, Behold, the bridegroom cometh; go ye out to meet him. Then all those virgins arose, and trimmed their lamps. And the foolish said unto the wise, Give us of your oil; for our lamps are gone out. But the wise answered,

saying, *Not so;* lest there be not enough for us and you: but go ye
rather to them that sell, and buy for yourselves. And while they
went to buy, the bridegroom came; and they that were ready
went in with him to the marriage: and the door was shut.
Afterward came also the other virgins, saying, Lord, Lord, open
to us. But he answered and said, Verily I say unto you, I know
you not. Watch therefore; for ye know neither the day nor the
hour wherein the Son of man cometh."

The Parable of the Talents:

"For *the kingdom of heaven is* as a man traveling into a far
country, *who* called his own servants, and delivered unto them
his goods. And unto one, he gave five talents, to another two,
and to another one; to every man according to his several
ability; and straightway took his journey. Then he that had
received the five talents went and traded with the same, and
made *them* other five talents. And likewise he that *had received*
two, he also gained other two. But he that had received one went
and digged in the earth, and hid his lord's money. After a long
time the lord of those servants cometh, and reckoned with them.
And so he that had received five talents came and brought other
five talents, saying, "Lord, thou deliver unto me five talents:
behold, I have gained beside them five talents more." His lord
said unto him, "Well done, *thou* good and faithful servant: thou
hast been faithful over a few things, I will make thee ruler over
many things: enter thou into the joy of thy lord." He also that
had received two talents came and said, "Lord, thou deliver
unto me two talents: behold, I have gained two other talents
beside them." His lord said unto him, "Well done, good and
faithful servant; thou hast been faithful over a few things, I will
make thee ruler over many things: enter thou into the joy of thy
lord." Then he which had received the one talent came and said,
"Lord, I knew thee that thou art a hard man, reaping where
thou hast not sown, and gathering where thou hast not strewed:
and I was afraid, and went and hid thy talent in the earth: lo,
there thou hast *that is* thine." His lord answered and said unto
him, "*Thou* wicked and slothful servant, thou knewest that I
reap where I sowed not, and gather where I have not strewed:
thou oughtest therefore to have put my money to the

exchangers, and *then* at my coming I should have received mine own with usury. Take therefore the talent from him, and give *it* unto him, which hath ten talents. For unto every one that hath shall be given, and he shall have abundance: but from him that hath not shall be taken away even that which he hath. And cast ye the unprofitable servant into outer darkness: there shall be weeping and gnashing of teeth."

Pastor Rob Thomas, why did you hide the one talent I gave you in the earth? Why when I told you my heart's cry, that I could do nothing in the earth unless you pray. But you and your filth that stood in my house, and sold that one talent as on the days, that you reserved for united prayer you held bible training courses in the ways of that false prophet Jezebel as you taught about the gifts of the Holy Spirit, while my children lay dying in the streets as I grieved, watching you and others like Bishop Peter Jakes, selling what I said I gave freely so that no man can boast for it is a free gift. Have you not read **Ephesians 2:8-9, "For by grace are ye saved through faith; and that not of yourselves: *it is* the gift of God: not of works, lest any man should boast. For we are his workmanship, created in Christ Jesus unto good works, which God hath before ordained that we should walk in them."**

Yes my true servant the apostle Paul did mention, that you do have the right to make a living of my word. But my word is the word of reconciliation and not of division, which is what you and your other Jezebel priest practice in my house of prayer. You write books and make commerce from my death, on the cross. I died for all not just a select few as you divide my children, for am I not the Father of all spirits but yet you write doctrines of hate and spew out of your mouth like the vomit of those who I have sent you to save from hell as they vomit up your false doctrines, which you call theology that you spend over 40,000 pounds to get when my children are lying dying from hunger in your own streets, paved with the blood of my true servants of long ago, who died trying to save these poor souls and so I brought revival so may times. Look at your misguided facts about the Muslims. Did I say that my gospel is the gospel of division and lies? I said it is the gospel of reconciliation and not by making them feel like the filth that you are as I saw you and you other prophets of the woman called Jezebel as you stood on the stage in Action, and he gave the story of the man who was judged, because he would not repent of his fornication, and then you gave the alter call, and they came up terrified of my judgments, revealing their shame to you as you fed, on their private shame as you force them to tell the whole world, what they did in secret, and then you insult my intelligence, thinking that I am blind, by putting in your statement purpose, that none of your leaders are involved in fornication, and then you ask on your bible school application form my poor wounded treasures to admit their shame, by telling you, if they were in pornography, when it is written that I will remember their sins no more.

Then why do you remind them of it as you dance like a filthy dog in my house? And then when you come together to pray what do you ask me for is not to deny another group, hence the gay community, their human dignity, thinking that I am the same God that you teach about on your platform as you celebrate what your grandfathers did to the Muslims in the Holy Crusades as you celebrate what they did in your foolish speeches, like your brothers the Politicians and remember what they did and are well known for as you watch on channel four the programs about the history of Christianity as the reporter began to show you what you are in my house of prayer as you think you will do once more do with your witchcraft literature, about how the Muslims are taking over England, remember what he said remember who he quoted it from and that was from the diaries of the Beast themselves, 'we killed young boys who were Muslims and then boiled them and consumed them.' And is this what you think I am, and yet you will not condemn these acts of cannibalism but promotes them in my house. Are you saying that no one has the right to live but by what you think, I am? And I ask you how much did the two pieces of wood and the four nails cost, that nailed me to the cross so that all could come to me?

And how much commerce did you accumulate, while I laid dying on the cross, bleeding to death, from a broken heart as the Father showed me you in this day but yet I saw what you would do as I hang there dying, and I said Father forgive them for they know not what they do. And the Father showed you what you are as in my deformed body on the cross as I died in agony, for those who you now deceive, saying that I am a God who will deny another group of people their rights as human beings, to choose whether I am a good God and not some monster, who is always condemning others in my name, which you have taken in vain Pastor Rob Thomas and Pastor Roy James. Now you know why you lost the building that I gave you in Action. Do you remember my watchmen as she came up to your platform, where you act out your fantasy of being me and I showed you your heart as she placed a coin by your feet, and your body guards jumped up ready to throw her down to ground, and drag her screaming from your filthy presence as you idealized what you thought was my anointing, when I told you through, my servant Smith Wigglesworth as he departed from this earth, "My glory I will not share with another." Who do you think I was talking about? And remember it was Roberts Smith that I told to make a record of why some of my generals failed and why some made it, and you did not understand who I was talking about. And when I sent one of my watchmen to Smith Wigglesworth, to test his heart, what did he say that is the watchman? He said, 'what is the secret of your power?' and what did Smith Wigglesworth say? Did he not say, 'A broken and contrite heart I will not despise?'

Tell me Pastor Rob Thomas is your heart contrite and broken before me? And if it is not, then what do you think that I think of you? And you Roy James you talk about my past glory as if you know me but when I come to you in the form of my watchmen, to test your heart so that you can see what you really are in my presence, what do you call me. As your servants, the ushers tells my watchmen to be quiet, while they are obeying me, and that is praying for did I not say my house shall be called a house of prayer but you make it a den of thieves as you sell my grace, yes remember pastor Rob Thomas, when you wrote your obituary in my servant Wendy Jones' book called, 'I was no prophet?' Then did you not see what I said about those who turn my house into a place of business offering courses that you can take for free at any college? What did I say and you wrote your name on my holy word, to bring fame to yourself but you did not think, because if you look at the title, 'I was no prophet,' that was my message to you, to warn you that I knew what you were going to do. Hence, you are no prophet of mines. I said you cannot serve two masters. You cannot serve God and mammon, why did you not listen? As you, admire yourself in my house? When I got up in anger and left, did you not say I was a devil, and

Horace Smith

that I was mad, and the whole audience who say they love me began to laugh at me as I left? And then the next evening you are preaching about the Good Samaritan. Therefore I will remind of you of my words, 'whoever sins against the Holy Spirit, his sins will not be forgiven.' That is to call his work the work of the devil. Therefore, I will encourage you to repent, before the day of the vengeance of the Lord comes. And then you pastor John where does it say in my word, that you can force those who are poor in my household to go and borrow from Social Welfare, a thousand pounds each, to feed your greed? And then answer me this one question do you think I am really that blind?

I saw when you told my treasure either marry you or leave the church, I saw when you sent the spirit of death to slay pastor Rob Thomas, and then in your fake smile you said as if it was my Holy Spirit to pray that he does not die, that is pastor Rob Thomas, do you think I was blind, when you sent your angels to kill his daughter instead when I prevented you from murdering him? Do you think I am blind when you have those who are poor take out loans much more than they can pay back to build that cloth tent that you call my house. And when you began to work them like the dog that you are what did I tell you as my watchman came to you in horror, and said that is enough as her husband built your egotistic pride to your Goddess Jezebel as he almost collapsed from the exhaustion of your folly.

Did I not say all those who are heavy burden come to me, and I will give you rest? Then is that what you call rest in my kingdom pastor John? And then do you think I was blind, when you told your Lord and master the fool that sit on the throne above London to move, and then you boast in your foolish wit as you said in my name Jesus to his throne move and it moved. When I said before I went to my Father in heaven that those who believe in my name shall cast out demons, heal the sick, speak new languages, take up serpents, and if they drink any poison it will not hurt them, then which Jesus moved the prince of this country's throne, and remember, before you see your folly in the deeper workings of Satan, my spiritual champion Elijah saw it all, and he was shocked asking me did I do that, because not even Elijah, my trusted servant have I ever asked me to move a throne, and then the question is this why would I? What

If I Am Then I Must Be

would be the point? Would a fallen angel's throne bring my people closer to me? And then we see what you did how many fell dead under your pastoral ministry. How many did you tell me to kill, while you were in Jamaica, because you could not get your own why?

When I told you through the apostle James that I cannot be, tempted with evil I am the prince of life, and not the bringer of death. And you, like all the false apostles, that came out of Africa, like the cowards that you are will you pay back the loan that you had Peter Walters, and the treasure of mines to sign for? And what did you say to my watchman Horace James Barrocks, and it is not Smith it was Satan that changed his last name to Smith, when he sodomized him at the tender age of ten to turn him into one of you but he remained faithful, even unto death of his own soul. And remember you Satanist, murdered five of his family, cut off his niece legs that was only five at the time, and left her brain dead, and blind. Remember my words are true vengeance is mines, I will repay it is called, 'the Day of the Lord,' so I will cry out to you to repent of this madness, that I would give sinful man, my glory as you think I have given you. As you sent your assassins to cut of his niece feet and leave her blind, murdering three of his brothers, then telling him as I watched you that you do not care about him and the devil, or how about you do not have the time to waste helping one of my dying treasures, you remembered how you would look at him with disgust in your heart.

It was me that you were despising in him. And then remember, before I gave you Big Lane and you taught your false doctrines, that is the deeper works of Satan, you look right into his soul, and you saw me looking right back at you and you knew that I saw the coldness of your heart, and how much you really despise me, and yet you rob the poor with false promises saying that I am restoring Mount Zion, when I never said that I said to Peter who do you say I am and he replied that I am the son of God, and I told him that flesh and blood did not reveal this unto him it was God and upon that Rock I will build my church, and the gates of hell shall not prevail. What is that Rock? It is Horace James Barrocks, hence the Rock, and Bar as in Barjona, hence Jonah the sign that I said I would give this generation that is the preacher of righteousness, and not restoration. Did you not read Psalm Chapter 15, when you meet these requirements, then you will abide in my tabernacle. And then pastor John, I beg you please explain to me where, when I walked the earth, when did I actually grew back flesh on a crushed hand as you thought I did to you, when your Father that is Satan, the devil crushed it in your car door, and you went to the bathroom to wash of the blood and you saw the flesh growing back, then in your falseness, you ran out of the bathroom, trying to deceive my children at what you lied to them, that I was doing. I will encourage to go and read the book that I had my true servant, 'Mary Baxter,' write called, 'Divine Revelation of Hell,' go to the chapter were I showed Satan in his private chambers, and the witches, that had died and gone to hell, and now they serve him on the earth as the walking dead, what did he do to them, to warn them not to fail him as they seduced my children into the deeper workings of his kingdom. Did he not cause snakes and other vile creatures to come out of their flesh as a warning, that he would expose them, if they failed? Is not that the same sign that you tried to convince my servant Elijah that that vile magic trick, that you did was from my Spirit and remember what I said, while I walked the earth that calling the work of the Holy Spirit the work of devils I will not forgive, and then pastor John, you boast, that you have a daughter at Harvard university is this right? How come she has never visits you in London? And if she really existed, what is she saying to you as her own father? And when you said that you divorced your first wife did you show your second wife your divorce papers?

Remember I said you will know them by their fruits so where is your fruits of righteousness pastor John? Such as love, joy, longsuffering, faith, gentleness, temperance, peace, goodness, gentleness, meekness? Why your fruit is found in the works of the flesh as in the Homo erectus, the primitive species that you are. Go and watch the mind of your husband Jezebel as she appeared on the screen as Doctor Manhattan and remember my champion battled her face to face and you saw what he saw when you look at the poster of the advert of one of Will Smith in the movie, 'I am Legend,' look at how she described my champion, in the intense heat of that one encounter look at how resolute his face was as the weapons of warfare are used and remember that was just one encounter with her and his instruction from his true king and Lord, me was to just restrain her and do not hurt her. There is no repentance in the grave only judgment. And you know yours already. And you Ankle, you proclaim that I am a God that, if you worship me, the blessings will come down. Are you saying that I bless the filth that you call worship? Or are you saying that I am a whore like your wife, that you breed, like the whore you married, and when I show you what you really are and they are those who you say you are sick of swearing in your church and notice they use the word like fuck then you know I am the discerner of the thoughts of the hearts, for I created them and am I not showing you yours, and your other whoring Balaam worshippers get up in my house, and say that you are sick and tired of them swearing in the house of the Lord, and then you and the other Homo erectus species of worshippers, that say they love me to call on the blood of my risen son to curse them when it was shed for their sins by pleading it as you run around my house screaming like when you are making love to the cow that you call your wife, and remember I am also the creator of the faces of all human beings and don't you think I created the whore that you married to look like a cow to show you your true heart as I reveal it to you, saying that as you praise me the blessings come down and consider this, if I am a whore like your true mother, that harlot the Mystery Babylon, then look at how much I think of your worship you are bus boy in a restaurant is that my blessing?

Then why would you call me a holy God a whore that blesses lip service, and remember what is written in my word the incenses of my true worshippers that go up to me, well just image yourselves as you are taking a shit in the morning when you wash your filthy mouths out with toothpaste after calling the Holy God of all ages, a God who blesses immorality that is practice in my house, just smell that shit, it is how your worship of me smell like, in my presence, be warned you worshippers of the doctrine of Balaam, I gave you time to repent, I will not wait much longer. As I said, "Rend your hearts before me not your garments. For it is written if my people who are called by my name will humble themselves and turn from their wicked ways I will hear from heaven and forgive their sins and heal their land." And you pastor Jack when I came to you as my watchman, and he asked you for a written reference, what did you write? Was it not he is a member of your whoring den of iniquities but however you will not help him financially. But yet you tell me that I must come to your bible school, and listen to the filth and lies that you teach with your Doctorate of Theology, when there is no such word in my Holy word. Then which doctrine are you teaching my sheep? And when, if I was there in your midst, why are not the sick healed, and why are you not healed. Remember when I told my watchman to lay hands on you and he prayed for you in your bell house, and what did he ask you was it not did you feel the anointing? And you said no what was he trying to tell you. I know those who are mines, and would I not have healed you, if you were my own child like your wife?

Then my watchman who is not working buries his own brother in my house, and you charge him for the use of my hall, and where was the keyboard player? Remember what my faithful servant your wife said to you? "He is a member of my house, do not take the forty pounds and you gave it back?" Do you think I could not see into your heart, and how dark it is? Then if he was a member of your church why did you not visit him in the hospital, when your boyfriend Peter Scot told you? But if it was one of your own children, then would you have treated them the same, and if you did how would you feel about yourself as a father but yet you show me your true heart, and treat my little ones with contempt, thinking I will not take your name and you whole whoring church of devils and Baal worshippers out my book of life? I say be wise and repent, I do not require sacrifices it is a broken and contrite that I will not despise.

This is your last warning. And you Mrs. Whiteman is that what they teach on your theology training degree, that when your, I think it was your son was robbed of his mobile phone to call on my name to go and do evil to the one who took it, when I told you when I walked the earth to forgive your enemies, be good to those who use you, and if they ask for a item give them your cloak too. Could you image how my Holy Angels looked at me, and wondered can you actual read, what is written in my word, you illiterate heifer and how I watched Satan rejoice in hell as he waits for your filthy soul and remember they love Christians in hell, it is like a delicacy of holy meat to them as they feed on your rotting corpse as you burn in the lake of fire, and remember this word, 'forever,' why did you use the name of the Lord in vain?. Now you have your answer why I will not use you to save my lost ones. I warn you repent, and I will show you mercy on judgment day, when I judge your mother Beast gone to seed that is planted in your filthy hearts. As you call on me as a God to hurt those I love and died for, on the cross, for the filth that you call worship of a Holy God.

Therefore, you goat nations listen again to your judgments.

The Judgment of the Nations:

"When the Son of man shall come in his glory, and all the holy angels with him, then shall he sit upon the throne of his glory: and before him shall be gathered all nations: and he shall separate them one from another, as a shepherd divideth *his* sheep from the goats: and he shall set the sheep on his right hand, but the goats on the left. Then shall the King say unto them on his right hand, Come, ye blessed of my Father, inherit the kingdom prepared for you from the foundation of the world: for I was a hungered, and ye gave me meat: I was thirsty, and ye gave me drink: I was a stranger, and ye took me in: naked, and ye clothed me: I was sick, and ye visited me: I was in prison, and ye came unto me. Then shall the righteous answer him, saying, Lord, when saw we thee hungered, and fed *thee? O*r thirsty, and gave *thee* drink? When saw we thee a stranger, and took *thee* in? Or naked, and clothed *thee?* Or when saw we thee sick, or in prison, and came unto thee? And the King shall answer and say unto them, Verily I say unto you, Inasmuch as ye have done *it* unto one of the least of these my brethren, ye have done *it* unto me. Then shall he say also unto them on the left hand, Depart from me, ye cursed, into everlasting fire, prepared for the devil and his angels: for I was a hungered, and ye gave me no meat: I was thirsty, and ye gave me no drink: I was a stranger, and ye took me not in: naked, and ye clothed me not: sick, and in prison, and ye visited me not. Then shall they also answer him, saying, Lord, when saw we thee a hungered, or athirst, or a stranger, or naked, or sick, or in prison, and did not minister unto thee? Then shall he answer them, saying, Verily I say unto you, Inasmuch as ye did *it* not to one of the least of these, ye did *it* not to me. And these shall go away into everlasting punishment: but the righteous into life eternal."

"If you will turn from your wicked ways, and pray I will hear from heaven, and forgive your sins, and I will heal your land but remember only if you turn from your wicked ways. That is what I called vile as your practice of your place to the idol Baal as you practice in my temple, a temple of prayer and worship, in truth and spirit." "But remember I am the Alpha and the Omega, and I know the end better than you know your beginnings as I told my servant, 'Ezekiel,' long ago." "But the house of Israel will not hearken unto thee; for they will not hearken unto me: for all the house of Israel *are* impudent and hardhearted."

Therefore, go to your perspective judgments found in Revelation chapters 2 to 3, look at your sins, that you have committed, and why you have been judged, then look at the qualifications to over turn your judgments. Remember many of you will not believe, that is fine. But be warned; hear what the Spirit has said to the church. For further reading read Watchman Nee' book called, 'Revelation,' this will give more information on why it happened.

Look at Revelation chapters 17 and 18, this is why it happened then go to 1st Corinthians 11: 24-32, this will help you understand what is about to unfold remember this is his mercy to save you from the lake of fire. And if you want to see what Satan is planning for you in that lake which is the second death then go see the movie called, 'Watchmen,' go to the scene where the psychopath is in prison and watch the carnage this is what he has in mind for you in the lake of fire. And that is for eternity. He knew he could not win that is why that horrid filth in the movie goes into the bedroom of one of his enemies crying saying it was all a joke, that is the personified image of Satan as he waits for the revealing of his Beast, hence the fictional character of Doctor Manhattan, look at the symbol on his forehead it is the, 'Mark of the Beast,' it is the letter, 'I,' meaning infinity. And remember he is a giant, hence the race of Nephlims as written in Genesis 6, that God destroyed, by flooding them to death as they grieved his heart at what they were doing to his creation. Remember you have been warned.

Remember the wages of sin is death. But the gift of God is eternal life. And it is free.

If I Am Then I Must Be

Chapter 29

But if you have discovered, that your colleagues, in the case of my mother, are not committed to the task at hand, that is the sincere welfare of a ten year old child, and that is to help that ten year old child, sincerely mature, into a growing adult, with all the attributes of a good life, starting of with nothing but his faith in good people, and the sincere care of the adult community but instead as they are, 'sheep in wolf,' clothing, preys on the innocent and virtuous, to corrupt them with their lies and cheap tricks of witchcraft and magic, in their satanic ritual ceremony, to make a vulnerable child into their host, like the Daemon story, that is so well played out on television, in the Omen saga.

It is so disheartening to discover from a parent's point of view, that your colleagues, the ones who you trusted your ten year old treasure to have no morals, are devastating, especially when you have been abused yourself. And my mother grew up in the church abused, she went from man to man, having children, like their own private little whore, because she in their eyes was a slag but in mines a trusting old soul, that was abused and left broken hearted, her children from her previous relationships turned against her, and then to see three of her precious treasures die two murdered and the other one bled to death as his spleen ruptured, because he was drinking himself to death, to prove, like all men, that he was a man but deep inside he was crying out for help, for someone to love him and so subconsciously, by drinking himself to death, he thought that he would be saved, in time but the truth was that the hero, that you see in the fantasy films, coming in from the north to save the day is what it is in the films, a fantasy, a trick of the eyes, to convince those who are slow at heart, that escapism is the way to go. Just spend about forty pounds, for the whole family to go and be their fantasy, for one evening and just forget about your real lives, which are falling apart, and just go into the dubbing dream land of the fantasy of the hero complex, and so they wait for that knight in shinning amour to come and save them but in truth, he never comes and they wait until they are too old to wait anymore and so they take the next best thing. A man who has a good career and can bare children so that they can look like happy families, when in fact they still believe the lie, that was told to them in the Cinderella fairy tale of the slut bag who was fighting against two other slut bags to win the affection of, 'Prince Charming,' who turned out to be a true illusion, because no one is that perfect as my mother has learnt through fifty heart gut wrenching years as she was the wench for the filthiest of beasts, they call themselves real men when they are in truth but boys trying to be men. And then because each betrayal results in a broken heart and a deeper wound that cannot be healed, because I trusted these evil religious men, who thirst for power, to a point that they destroyed all that was good in me. I am still haunted by the image of what they were as they compared it to the image of what they had become.

The sense of lost is so great, when someone conceals the truth but when that truth is finally revealed, it makes you feel empty. Because you know that, you have lived a lie, based on your own perception of your illness and that is why it did happened to me, in my case. But I am not saying that every one who suffers from mental illness thinks, the same way. No, I am saying that this is the way I use to think about my illness until through therapy at SLAM and Cooltan Arts and Mosaic Clubhouse, has taught me, that I am human and that I can live a great life, living with mental illness, in the community, with the breakthroughs that, the Labour Party has made through their kind and compassionate debates, though they seem very boring as I watch them on the Parliament Channel. And this concept drove me to attempt suicide and the reason why, because what I thought it was the truth. And the truth was in fact a shadow on the ground, a dark picture of the colour black, that kept on moving in the light, I could not identify what it was, because it had no real shape just like the act of sodomy, it was a shadow, that I was trying to create from an fantasy like those who go to the movies, to escape the realism of their mundane lives.

I tried to reconstruct the act of sodomy and in so I created my illness. But many mental health practitioners will not agree with me, because they are too scientific in their analyst of the disease. So I am left alone, again to fathom the mysteries of this disease called mental illness, in a spiritual context. While they go on to live, their lives I am stuck with the mammoth task of coming to terms with a shadow so I came to the conclusion, after 18 years of therapy that I should learn to have fun. And learn to love myself, for who I am and not what society wants me to be. And that is a successful hero type of a man, well groom, that I am but I am no hero.

My and your world becomes stricken with a disease of the heart, it is called Fear, and that is not to trust anyone again so I live the lives of fears and woe, in fantasies and nightmares as I torment my anguished soul by trying to create the shadows and give them life when they do not exist in me. But however, what I have come to realize is that it was all a lie, a representation of man's inhumanity to man. As I look on and reflect on my shadows that will not come to life but not religion for religion is mind control and religion makes you an inhuman machine, like the Terminator, Hollywood's ideal of the church throughout its history, who are willing to destroy and murder in the name of God, what they cannot control or understand, that is me. But my faith was in a relationship with the Lord Jesus Christ, seeing him as another person, like me who I could talk to and would talk back to as a friend, a brother, and a father, a compassionate high priest that is Jesus who would always talk back to me in his conscience. And I learnt one more very important life lesson about my illness, and that was my anger at what had happened as I watched my fury in the kick ass movies, that I saw at the cinemas, was based on an ideal, that man could be God and have power or control over the weak and vulnerable. Like me at the age of ten. When Henry and Harry sodomized me and destroyed what I thought was my life but my life had not begun, I was in the process of learning about life so that I could live it more effectively.

It is like learning a career what do you learn to transgress you through the world of business in my case I was learning what it would take me to transgress through life, and not end up on the road to nowhere. For they thought an idea, that many have died in conflicts for since the day man first began to walk the earth, like Cain and Abel, and if this idea had any truth to it, this idea would have succeeded in controlling the hearts and minds of every one on the face of this earth. This idea would have brought healing, prosperity for all and much more but all it has done is to bring death and destruction from century to century without end, also known as for me a kind of mental illness, that I will have for the rest of my life. In my case, it is called schizophrenia. The doctors say it is an incurable disease of the mind but to me it an unforgivable idea of the mind, because mental illness is like a cloak of evil spirits, who are parasites, feeding of your fears. And to heal myself, I have to find peace, which I already have peace and so I was never ill in the first place, because illness is the absents of peace, hence peace removed from one's self mind, emotions and feelings, which leads to the development of psychotic illnesses, which in my case is called schizophrenia, an illness that is thought up from the shadows of the past, until it has taken form in the mind, the real of perception.

It is called the blue print to the home that you are making for yourself, which in therapy for 18 years have brought down as to build a near perfect structure called serenity, peace and much creativity. By the forgiveness of myself for allowing it to happen then I am totally and completely healed and well and cured but the doctors cannot accept that I am well and can be cured from what their scientist said is an incurable disease and if I was to argue with them over the subject they would write in my notes that I am displaying psychotic episodes of delusions that I am well when in truth there is no cure from a disease that scientist say cannot be cured, and the amazing thing about their presumption is that it is based on evidence that has been recorded as the outward manifestation of the disease, because in truth mental illness is of the hidden mind, and not the visible mind so what is seen is from the hidden part of the illness, and that is where the illness is conceived by the patients' conviction, that he or she is unwell when in fact they have developed a different way of seeing life, that is scary to them and to the scientist so instead of developing new ways of expressing themselves, they are probed to find out what this new way of seeing is, and so classify it as a psychotic episode, and so assign them to the prison of mental illness, and because they reawakening to this thing called life without conscience as the humanist would put, 'there is no God so enjoy yourself,' hence the ethos of what Hitler did with his Nazi Germany that killed so many and created some of the more horrid ways of expressing what is hidden in the dark deep recesses of the shadow of one's fallen ego, the id as in the, 'Oedipus Complex,' as developed by Freud. But however, for them to accept that they are in fact wrong in a broad sense they would have to see that something is wrong with all their years of study and the ideology of Freud who divulged the secrets of

If I Am Then I Must Be

Hitler's and Stalin's minds and their comrades in arms as they murdered and killed for their sexual fantasies as we are taught about the deeper works of the Satanists. And yes, murder and in this case mass murder as in Mass is the last stage of the disease called sexual fantasy. It is when you have broken all your conscience conviction of the concept of true love and that is to love just one person all your life as we pronounced on your wedding day in the ceremony that joined two people that love each other together for life.

However, when this law, planted by God, in the conscience of man for our own protection is violated, then love becomes lust and lust turns into sexual desire and sexual desire turns into boredom and boredom turns into sexual perversion and sexual perversion turns into obsession and obsession turns into if I cannot have you then no one can and then, the end, which is a complete breakdown of all the laws of the conscience, that stops the moral decay of a society as we saw Europe so fast turned into a amoral decadence, during World War II, where sexual fantasies became sadistic murder as we saw in the death camps. The impetus there is evil as an active force, released by psychopathic behaviour. The main example would be the influence of Streicher, who derived sexual gratification from the persecution and torture of helpless people. There is no doubt that thousands of similar characters were attracted to membership of the SS by similar prospects. But it is equally certain that they were a small minority among all those involved in the Holocaust. Page 89 Hitler and Nazi Germany by Stephen J. Lee ISBN 0-415-17988-2-9-780415-179881

Chapter 30

A wanton star, without restraint or inhibition and done out of desire, heedless of the, 'Law of Caused and Effect,' commonly known as Karma, the eastern philosophy to which the quality of your past life determines your current and future life, which someone, an unsuspecting fool has already lived, for all roads lead to Rome, that is called a place going to nowhere on the road to nowhere The Holy Roman Empire, that became the United States of Europe, that Hitler tried to purge to create his genetically perfect race of Supermen, that Napoleon tried to conquer, and two world wars fought on her soil, it is called your chosen destiny, the path that you take in life, what you sow you reap or what you sow you inherit as your reward for all that is done by oneself to oneself in the mirror of consciousness, the mirror of life, reflected backwards in time, our unions with each other as we try to change each other's perceptions, to our own way of thinking, thus changing ourselves, by creating an image of our desires in our relationships with others, some try to change what they hate in what they consider to be a good friend, whispering sweet words of lustful passion to feed their desires, into the ear of this friend, a sweet lullaby.

A gentle song to sooth a child, to a conscious sleep and when that friend falls asleep the change begins, and so the Frankenstein monster begins to awake from the id, the hidden desires of the darkness, and as the changes takes hold so does the beholder of the change begin to see his creation come alive but not in his friend but in himself for his friend is a reflection of hidden dreams, visions, even fantasies and even nightmares and so he only sees an illusion, simply called the wishful thinking, just like a tree has not changed in the six thousands years that a tree has existed so it is with the human heart for it is desperately wicked and what is evil it will do, but as a wise Rabbi said to a blind Rabbi, "Verily, verily, I say unto thee, Except a man be born again, he cannot see the kingdom of God." The blind Rabbi replied, "How can a man be born when he is old? Can he enter the second time into his mother's womb and be born?"

The wise Rabbi replied, "Verily, verily, I say unto thee, except a man is born of water and of the Spirit, he cannot enter the kingdom of God. That which is born flesh is flesh; and that which is born of the Spirit is Spirit. Marvel not that I said unto thee, ye must be born again." The blind Rabbi now completely confused and bewildered asked again, "How can these things be?" Then the sweet sound of the winds of unconsciousness, the hidden echoes of intuition, whispers into the eternity of his heart the words of the ancient seer Isaiah, "Who hath believed our report? And to whom is the arm of the Lord revealed? For he shall grow up before him as a tender plant, and as a root out of a dry ground: he hath no form nor comeliness: and when we shall see him, there is no beauty that we should desire him.

He is despised and rejected of men; a man of sorrows, and acquainted with grief: and we hid as it were our faces from him; he was despised, and we esteemed him not. Surely, he hath borne our grief: and carried our sorrows: yet we did esteem him stricken, smitten of God, and afflicted. But he was wounded for our transgressions, he was bruised for our iniquities: the chastisement of our peace was upon him; and with his stripes we are healed." As the man who continues to look into the mirror of perception, is by changing his friend, he changes himself, for it is only his perception in the mirror of his conscience that changes and it is only awareness, that comes alive as he becomes aware of the darkness of his soul as he runs from the sound, the sweet sounds of the winds of unconsciousness, the hidden echoes of intuition, as what was known from the beginning is frown up, in the displeasure of the facial expression of communication of the intellect, 'If I am I must be,' and when consciousness came alive in these words, "And the Lord God formed a container for consciousness from the dust of the ground, and breathed into his nostrils the wind of intuition and consciousness became a living soul knowing everything, and continues to whispers into the eternity of his heart," "Why don't you remember," and how unhappy he really has become with his miserable life, because he refuses to remember, and thus in the word, 'If I am I must be' and so he is and so he becomes, as he thinks he is, as with a wise king of the ancient days once wrote 'For as he thinketh in his heart, so is he.' As the Wright Brothers thought, they were birds and so they became birds in their mechanical flying machine and the Ford as he thought he could outrun a Jaguar and so he became a mechanical automobile. As the seeds of evolution from Darwin's tree of life began to spring up, where William Shakespeare once began his journey, 'If I am then I must be,' and as like we cannot see the routes of the natural tree, how it is formed, how it grows, and what it is becoming, until it is what it has become, and that is visible, a tree, we cannot see the route of the theoretical tree of life of Charles Darwin but only in our thoughts as Shakespeare thought these words, "There is nothing either good or bad but thinking makes it so." And I watched her in college as she told me how she hated the church and that they were fake people, not sincere, not realizing that she was using her hatred for Christians to describe herself.

In so inheriting hate, adultery, fornication, uncleanness, lasciviousness, idolatry, witchcraft, variance, emulations, wrath, strife, seditions, heresies, envying, drunkenness, revelling, which leads to murder and then the end of her journey to Rome, via the Lake Of Fire, that burns with Brimstone and sulphur forever and forever, thus the Frankenstein monster breathes and awareness, 'If I am then I must be,' comes and this monster, the id, comes alive in her heart, as we have seen in so many past generations that has destroyed the world over and over like the, 'Ground Hog Day,' scenario, being repeated forever and ever, or more commonly known as the psychological make up Homo sapiens, the mask he wears to entice those who are blind and cannot see

For it was she that said I would sit on his face referring to a young golden black prince that she lusted after in college. As she brings her fantasy to life from the seed of thoughts giving him cunnilingus oral stimulation of her genitals using his tongue and lips to stimulate sexual pleasure and desire. It was she that told me many times that she would invite me to her home for a barbecue with the others members of our class, it was she that spoke behind the backs of the Africans in our class, calling them stupid and ignorant and so it was she, who she was creating in her id, thus giving life to the Frankenstein monster within her, to be finally revealed to the world as the modern woman. Her name is Diana. And in the realm of perception of our own reflection as a wise man wrote, "And, behold I come quickly, and my reward is with me, to give every man according as his work shall be. Surely, I come quickly. He that is unjust, let him be unjust still, and he which is filthy, let him be filthy still, and he that is righteous, let him be righteous still, and he that is holy, let him be holy still," the provocation to the reflection of our perception as it forms vaguely in the light of our id the source of our primitive instincts and drives and the cause of anger as the darkness engulfs the light of our perceptions of our own reflections, in the mirror of ourselves reflected in life. One man's meat is that he sees his own skin colour as a reflection in the mirror of his small little world in the skin of another man alien from his own and because that man's skin colour is a darker shade of his own, he is able to express his true feelings about his own self hidden in the secret place of the id, which according to Freud is theoretical or theatrical part of his human hidden conscience as he acts out his performing role in his play on the stage of the world as one famous president resounded as he was interviewed by the witnesses of time, "History will tell if I have made the right decision, to go to war," and where the opaque blackness, that old serpent of darkness hides as he beguiles us to eat the forbidden fruit of conscience, the legendary and mythical green apple the envy of the modern world, and despicable and so forms, in the light of his perception, a reflection of his interpretation of his own feelings about himself in another darker man's skin, as he spews hate and abuse, which leads to great suffering, misery towards the object, that the light is reflected of a *black* man so creating a mirror for him to look into to dress himself in the morning, putting on his make up, washing his face, brushing his teethes, combing his hair, to look like a God, the Homo sapiens, and so he travels the destiny of a racist and a bigot, until he reaches Rome. The Holy Roman Empire, a creation of the collective imagination, the soul of consciousness, a faded memory of a once powerful empire, that rule most of the world with brutality and violence.

Yes an ideal, a thought of the imagination, that came alive and breathe upon the world, its fiery breath of destruction as she shed the blood of the innocent, in the satanic mad aim, to make the whole Barbarian world civilize, a reflection of the Holy Roman Empire, thus functioning as Gods and making life a so call son in the tradition of God creating his first son, a living, breathing soul from the dust, Adam, and then his second son, a quickening spirit Jesus, as the small inward voice of the conscience of Rome is heard in the intuition of Rome saying, "Give me children," then becomes a cry then a loud yell until it becomes, the never ending cries of the Gods, Apollo, Mars. But in the process created her, the Frankenstein monster, as she projected what she really was, in her God conscience onto other civilizations as she stuck out at anything that reminded her of her.

And so she creates the past hatreds and strife of ages gone past, in the future and so the fruit from the tree of knowledge good and evil is consumed, by another generation doomed to repeat the past as the old saying, 'the past always repeats itself,' like a living organism, that cannot die, because we won't let it die as we create our dislikes and what we hate about ourselves in our reflection in the mirror of conscience as we enter the Holy city of Rome. Another man sees what somebody or a something is called, a word, a term, a phrase that distinguished an honoured guest separating them from the others in his mirror of perception, reflected back at him as he is observed from far away and is seen to have seen the face of hope the face of Aegus looking out yonder into the red the perception of red, the deep blue emotions, and as the seed from Charles Darwin's Tree Of Life begins to sprout into a tiny little tree the deep blue emotions takes of the species of tree, in the form of guilt, pity, regret, depression, remorse, and it continues to grow into a beautiful tree spouting its green leaves of envy as it sways in the winds of the hopelessness, its now tall brown trunk is its foundation, its begin to take shape and it identity is known of what species of tree it is and from what family of trees it came from and it is identified as coming from the family of the trees of Oedipus.

A religious devotion to ones own ego, the strong respectful devotion to the deity of self-belief, and the strict observance of the egotist the Oedipus complex, a Greek mythological figure a son of Jocasta and Laius, King of Thebes, who unwittingly killed his father and married his mother. And then being an egotist he puts out his own eyes, when he discovered what he had done. Like Hitler, blowing out his brains, when he realized what he had done, because of his ego. Later to be known as the Oedipus Complex, a theory from the mind of Sigmund Freud, who discovered by eating the forbidden apple from the Tree of the Knowledge of Good and Evil, the unconscious desire for parent's feelings and desires originating from when a child, more commonly a son unconsciously seeks sexual fulfillment from the parent of the opposite sex as he sees his son's ship returning home all with black sails hoisted. Thus now perceiving the colour red as the opaque black, the vine of the Oedipus Complex, the darkness is coming thinking that his cherished son had died Aegus hurls himself into the sea of forgetfulness, to be remembered no more but only in the dreams of the young who inspire to change what cannot be changed for death is a certainty and life a commodity, a traded item, an item that is bought and sold, especially like raw materials or even manufactured items that are for sale in the auction of understanding, as the end of the 18 years of the Tories auctioning government, a new error herald in as change comes in priorities from a government whose policies enslaved the living to the market forces of a government with a social conscience, which improve people's lives.

Then in five months time, a new auction of the understanding is announced by the Observer, the editor, Will Hutton, as inspired by the taste of the fruit from the Darwin's Tree Of Life called logic, and reasoning wrote "That those who think the market should not be left to devastate lives unchecked face, 'the growing realization that we may soon not be able to look to the Labour Party to represent what we believe." Then one of the auctioneers John Edmonds the general secretary of the GMB, creates being, by writing in January 1998, "Working people should be looking forward to 1998 as the best year in two decades. Yet, as I go around the country, what I find is not joyous expectation but a mood of gloomy cynicism." And it is announced, Labour has come the fruit called. 'on the right; Labour' the new Labour, a correlation with trade, and with the commerce, that is the Egyptian empire of trade and commerce as the great, great, great, grand parents of the Jews well know, unifying all, and the opportunities for that thing called a leftist revival should Labour fail to serve the luscious pieces of fruit, that Tony Blair had promised, is now for sale. As his marketing strategy is revealed Thatcher had consumed the fruit of, 'If I am then I must be,' and in so prunes the tree of the interpretation of perception, from the family of the Tree of the Knowledge of Good and Evil, that is mirrored back at us, in our id, the dark recesses of the soul, thus changing the understanding of the face of British politics, the face we see staring back at us, that is our own awareness of our alter ego

Clark Kent and Karl El, that is the light refracted by the bending of the light of the perception of understanding, that consumers were now more conservative.

Hence Labour policies reflected a shift. Labour' the modernization of the fruit of perception from Darwin's Tree Of Life, is now ripe for the auction, was an currency of the background, that prince charming' elections depended on the alluring Middle England, and that policies of denationalization or tax and spend would alienate Labour from the hurling into the sea of forgetfulness, to be remembered no more but only to live on in the dreams of the young, who inspire to change what cannot be changed for death is a certainty and life a commodity, a traded item, an item that is bought and sold, especially like raw materials of human worth as they put men on the Moon, and search for life in the outer regions of space spending millions on developing technology, that builds their trade with the God of commerce Mammon, like the Israelites being forced to build the great ancient pyramids of the old world, that so many admire, not considering all the death, misery and hardship they caused in the development of the Homo sapiens, and from the grave the Pharaohs still make trade and commerce as tourist come and visit their monuments to the giants of capitalism, that lives on in our memory and dreams but yet do little or nothing for the starving millions, dying everyday from the heritage of their ancestors of the Homo sapiens, who went to their ancient worlds of colours and dance and robbed everything, that they could lay their hands to build the Western Empires of the world, or even manufactured items of man's pride, that are for sale in the auction of understanding, and so we come full circle and full circle and full circle as, 'Ground Hog Day,' is repeated forever and forever and Labour is still vomiting out its sales rhetoric and oratory in public speaking, speaking that communicates its point persuasively, a complex labyrinth of nouns, adjectives, pronouns, adverbs and verbs, paragraphs, sentences of influence, and influentially posing a poetic dance, asking a question for effectiveness knowing intuitively not to expect nor require an answer like a rhetorician, a rhetoric teacher who teaches the art of using language successfully, and believably, skilled at sophisticated, fine sounding speech still being dependent on the working class, that it has mismanaged to get elected into the spot light of history, the stage of the world, the Globe theatre of modern life. And through the white lands of social deprivation, a state of poverty as the people cry out, "Where have all the great leaders gone?" Being without adequate food, and shelter, and so the deprivation syndrome develops from the Frankenstein monster, into a the beast as all look upon and gaze at the splendour of the beast, now woman who was arrayed in purple and scarlet colour, and decked with gold and precious stones and pearls, having a golden cup in her hand full of abominations and filthiness of her fornication with the kings of the nations, in every generation.

And upon her forehead was a name written, MYSTERY, BABYLON THE GREAT MOTHER OF HARLOTS AND ABOMINATIONS OF THE EARTH, drunken with blood of the saints, and with the blood of the martyrs of the Lamb of God, the kingdom to come, the beast they gazed upon is not, and shall ascend out of the bottomless pit, and go into perdition: and they that dwell on the earth shall wonder, whose names were not written in the book of life from the foundation of the world, when the Lamb was slain, when they behold the beast, that was and is not and yet is and here is the mind, which has wisdom.

The seven mountains, on which the woman sits and there are seven kings: five are fallen, and one is, and the other is not yet come; and when he comes, he must continue a short space, and the beast that was, and is not, even he is the eighth, and is of the seven, and goes into perdition, and the ten horns, which thou sawest are ten kings, which have received no kingdom as yet but receive power as kings one hour with the beast. These have one mind, and shall give their power and strength unto the beast, and the beast crosses the fields of social and economic policy, and becomes the party shifted towards the welfare to work schemes, to aide the long -term young unemployable, back into work, by making the receipt of benefits, conditional on seeking work or on receiving training. As the beast in human form promises in the 1992 elections to upgrade child benefit and pensions, and to link future pension increases to rises in prices or earning, which ever were the highest mountain to climb were abandoned, and the weak, and vulnerable, the voiceless were devoured by the ferocious teethes of the beast as the kings of the nation increased gas and electricity prices for greed so as they go to Polydom, the Lake of Fire, they have a nice pension, in the Lake of

Fire, to sustain them, in their new utopia, copying the Egyptians Pharaohs with their foresight into building the ancient pyramids, knowing that one day many will come to gaze upon the knowledge of the beast, and they would pay as well, and movies would be made, books would be written, a nice little investment for their retirement, they thought.

The beast's belief in his own spin, that it was Middle England who voted, and therefore was crucial to New Labour or as Mandelson so ingenuously put it, "Without New Labour the Conservatives could have won again.". But however, according to Draper, the famous meeting with the beast on 22nd May at Downing Street was about more than the impending European summit, the revival of the Holy Roman Empire, being consumed with the idea of welfare reform, especially for single mothers. However, the kings of the nation touched on an important thought, and that the British economy was not going into a period of long growth.

It was suggested that the majority of the British public wanted real reform, which was difficult to accomplish, without eating into their profits, in their business affairs as they prepared to journey to Polydom. This ideological shift, the post - war consensus on Keyesianism had been chopped down by the mid 1970s with the onset of stagnant growth, and then recession crept into the trunks of the other trees, and so by 1973 oil prices arose, and unemployment arose for the applauses of the beast, and the awards were handed out as government accepted their awards, from the International Money Fund in the forms of loans. And so unbridled capitalism created inequality and insecurity, and shatters the traditional social bonds, and denied people, and even countries, the power to control their own destiny, and so the nightmare of the growing old, the seas that is afterwards named after him, Aegus is immortalized in the dreams of the Homo sapiens as the man who continues to look into the mirror of perception is by changing his friend he changes himself, for it is only his perception, in the mirror of his conscience, that changes, and so it takes on another identity, it is only awareness, that comes alive as he becomes aware of the darkness of his soul as he runs from the sound, the sweet sounds of the wind of unconsciousness, the hidden echoes of intuition as what was known from the beginning is frown up, in the displeasure of the facial expression of communication of the intellect, 'If I am then I must be,' and when consciousness came alive, in these words, "Through faith also Sara herself received strength to conceive seed, and was delivered of a child, when she was past age, because she judged the Lord faithful who had promised." He was lost in the sea of forgetfulness for none can, when they enter Polydom, leave and so perception of the red, the deep blue emotions come alive in his soul of perception, in the mirror of reflection, without the light of perception for the darkness has come and will never go away, and so he is lost forever in the sea of forgetfulness, forgotten by the light of perception, a fading memory to the student of intellect as he makes his abode in the Lake of Fire for eternity. Where hope is dead and eternity is beginning.

Chapter 31

Therefore, my testimony of what I have been through comes into play but my life, a life, one of great sorrow and sadness that every one else can identify with, sodomized at the age of ten, by two Catholic priests, in a satanic ritual to make me the next conduit of the occults and the dark arts of the primitive. Moreover, in so knowing my life's story those who can see the light of this star will begin to hope again. First testimony John Knox second to none in all he suffered to live his life, the life that he wanted to live, under so much pressure and term oil. He was a Scots man, born 1514, and died 1572, he was the most unjustly despised, criticized, and hated of all the reformers of that day.

My second testimony of my life is president Cleveland who became president twice, simply in my eyes he told the truth that he had an affair, and fathered a child by another woman, just as I told the truth by letting the whole world know that I was sodomized by a satanic paedophile ring, at the age of ten, that lead to a thirty year love affair with pornography. I now see more clearly, the life giving spirit upon my life, in others. Moreover, I have noticed that many will condemn me for what they do in themselves, in secret Then Jane came into the room as I told Peter that I took the cat out for a walk, and the cat Joshua got lost, and could not find his way home. I thought, maybe he became too lazy. In addition, Jane began to look down on me as she screamed at me saying, "That is very a bad thing to do." If this had happened 20 years ago, I would have felt so much guilt.

However, I have grown by devoting my life to solitude, to discover my weaknesses, and to make my weaknesses my strength, and being condemned, by others is now one of my strengths. Therefore, it was like water of a duck's back, and that I really did not care about what she thought, even though I knew that she threw a chair at her mother, in a fit of rage. I had become a star, a spiritual star that brought hope to all those who intuitionally could see me, and knew that they were in darkness, that I had just finished my journey from, and those who were looking for the light, the door out of their darkness of sadness and sorrow, lost in a world of self-pity. Peter was astonished at Jane's comments, and spoke up abruptly saying, "That nothing is wrong with putting the cat out for semester."

Times were hard for my mother. She was illiterate, and in this world of woe, the academic colossal giant of humanity's goal to have a good understanding of what is past gone as in his story in history the story of man's conquest to monopolize humanity, like cattle in a cattle farm. Breeding only the strong and the fittest, the most intelligent are the only ones who are rewarded in this life of woe with beautiful whores, who spend all their time looking for a sucker a rich man, who they can live out their fantasy dream life, and their wild sexual fantasies. Missionary style, the 69 position, and the most perverse the fetish style of worship to the sex God Diana. Mum was not like that she was considered naïve, and because she was a lamb amongst wolves she was savagely destroyed, until now she live her life in endless regret and the sorrows of what could have been.

If she had stayed with my father Jasper, the jewel in her crown, he would have protected her and given her the dignity and security, respect she deserved. But through a cruel twist of fate she fell into the arms of a sexual predator who's only desire was to breed her like a whore then discard her with her children and not give them a penny in support, looking back he never gave me a penny of support either. However, he fed on my pure virtue, like a sodomite, on an innocent child as he rapes that innocent child repeatedly, in his perverted mind, that child for his perverse sexual gratification trying to make me like himself. I remembered how he would wash us, by wiping, rubbing us like something with light strokes, up and down, up and down, down in a plastic pale blue basin of hot soapy water. How disgusting it felt, and how I loathe such a horrid sexual act, in front of his siblings, who he did not care much for. He was an animal.

Then he would have us dance for him to amuse this fake shallow specimen of a man. I estimate in a loving relationship, a father can rub his child out of love, when cleaning that child. However, he was not my real father, and he certainly did not love me. So intuitionally, at that tender age, I know it was a lustful fantasy that he was living, in my fragile conscience. Maybe it reminded him how he touched my mother as his whore. Alternatively, how he touched other women, while he was with my mother that as he caught the clap from, and had to leave her, because my mother would no longer sleep with him. There is a line you do not cross with the poor. That is not to put their honour and godly pride to the test if you do it, it is war, and so he did cross that line.

He was a short mulatto skinned man, a taboo of both black and white ancestors, with short woolly hair. He worked for London Underground as a warden this was in the late 70s. In those days as I looked on in childlike eyes, his uniforms were very smart as I remembered it, a black coat and trousers, with a hat that looked like Hitler's Desert troopers that fought against Monty the python of the British Bull Dogs, the army of lions of the tribe of Judah. He would come home from work, and go into his room, and just sleep, and get drunk, like his oldest son Chester who he abandoned long ago as his words of blessings over his firstborn to the universe, when he was born to the world of woe and sorrows. "Give him up for adoption. He is no good and will come to nothing." In addition, his words came true. Chester did come to nothing. He committed suicide by drinking himself to death, hence rapture his spleen as he exited this world, in his little own rapture, in a small room in my mother's home. With me he spoke well maybe, I pleased him.

I remembered when he moved out of our rented home, when mum had come from work, I told her with elation the fucking prick was gone. However, I was very young then and it was before two Jamaican Catholic priest raped me. Therefore, my tongue was a tongue of an innocent child and not of a corrupt man as I am now. Who was obsessed with pornography, because of the church's stance of those who have been abused like me? That is to clean up your act, before you come into our church's community, and we will receive you. I was sodomized in a satanic ritual abuse ceremony. That began from my grandfather's side of family, when he made enemies in India, with those who were steeped and well verse in the arts of the occults. I was their goal to produce another Antichrist, a king of the arts in music, literature and the arts, then a great orator of the New Age ideology with demonstrations of the dark occults. Now it is called humanism formerly known as those great cities of Sodom and Gomorrah that Jehovah destroyed, in ancient times. She slapped me. I could not figure out why I now know that I am supposed to be her old age pension, her slave for eternity in this life, and the next. Maybe on an intuitive level I rebelled against everything that was inelegantly Jamaican and black, including her. I went to war to fight against any force that would try to make me a slave to religion, politics and a dead culture, when I am free, just to be and just to learn about life as a free black man who was white on the inside, like the freed Negro slave as he fought against his cultural practices of slavery. I learnt to hate my mother, then I learnt to love her, and then I learnt to pity her, in a good way. Not out of just blind pity. I even learnt to respect her, for what she went through, to raise her children. In addition, how many admired and came to her for guidance for she has the experience and has lived the life, and had survive its horrors. Then I learnt to forgive her for thinking, that I would lie down and die, to become her slave for eternity, and not my own free moral man. That I would not put up a fight, to break free from cultural practices, that leads to death, and woe and doom.

I was determined as I stood 22 years after my birth in the hospital called St, Thomas, were the flying bird from the loony tunes cartoons delivered me into the hardest battleground. The battleground of Humanism, because life to live, the life you want is a battlefield. As in the Song, 'Love is a battlefield.' In addition, the battle is simple, to find peace within yourself, without having to be apart of an institution like politic or religion, in a war of chaotic egos as all try to control the living making them the living dead. Peace then comes serenity, then a change in your perceptions, and you will begin to see all the colours, the rainbow that marked, and sealed the covenant God made with Noah, not to destroy the earth as man speeds up the process of the curse, in the earth and in my eyes the curse as written in Deuteronomy 28 is just going in the wrong direction, including Christianity, which I am a member of this club. Yes, God did make man in his own image, and one of the possessions he put into man is the ability to create. Like when humanism creates, HIV, cancer, death, wars, famine, economic greed, sexual perversion, bestiality and many more perverse forms of expressing the modern Homo sapiens, because laws and ideals cannot change the human heart, it must be born from above. Even in the church. Just look at the crusades, Henry the sixth, and even the witch burning ceremonies. I fought to the death against these ideological thinking patterns and forces, and won. I am now free to define my life, to choose who I associate with, what I study, what I listen to, and what I watch. I am not sentence to the fate of so many that are forced to serve a dead ideal, which is mind control as we saw in, 'Batman Begins.' The Bat is the image in dream symbolic symbols for witchcraft. But Hollywood puts it so elegantly. When Bruce Wayne's parents are killed, he blames himself, and so based on an ideal he becomes what he is now, a holy mother-fucking freak like Satan, decked out his black cape and fancy dress, that kills and murders to bring peace to his bat city, an avenging angle so to speak. Even though bat city has so many criminals, and many city officials are corrupted by greed. In the 1920s, in America, you had, 'Pretty Boy Floyd, AL Capone,' and many more. You had the, 'Italian Mafia,' you had corrupt city officials.

However, where are they today as they fade in the realm of nothingness, gone in a flash as so well put in Psalm 37, gone in a flash of an eye, yes now you have the, 'Latino and Afro American gangs.' However, if you keep teaching history as a present day thing, would you not live it repeatedly, until it destroys you? That was what my mother was trying to do to my life, and me destroying it, by not wanting me to grow up, and in so changing her limited perception of life, that is the ethos behind all cultures, to live the past in the present. If you look at the Jamaican diet, back then on the plantation, they needed that high starch diet to give them the energy to work the plantation fields but now those days are over, gone forever. But the Jamaicans still eat the same starchy foods as a celebration of the founding of the Jamaican people's dream of being a proud nations, of rich colours and food, which leads to all kinds of health problems, and so it is with all cultures as we look at another cultural people the Chinese' culture if you speak out against communism you are sentence to death. In a sense, it is like a prison, living on this earth. In addition, no one knows the way out. Even Christ had to die first, before he was let out of the prison of hopeless dreams, and never-ending nightmares, and then he had to appear to those who were trapped in the prison, wanting to escape, because many do not want to be freed from the prison of their conscience, look at Stalin. To show them the door and that is the way of the cross as we saw in the Passion of the Christ.

Chapter 32

We are inspired to be the same as we began as I remembered my father and always will. He was a kind and affectionate man. Dark skinned, his hair was all gone, and he cut the remaining bits regularly, at his local barbershop. His greatest wish was to see me have children so that he could enjoy the fruits of the labour that he did not work to produce in me.

The only words I ever heard from him as a child, that I remembered, were after a paedophile ring sodomized me, somehow he found out from other sources of what had happened. Maybe someone was going around taunting him, that I was gay. He came to see me that morning, this was the last time I would see him until I visited him from America. In addition, the last time that I would see him before I embarked on my journey to find what I had lost, that was my childhood, and my youth, and so in the process lost everything, and so gained nothing but woe, and sorrows, and endless regrets of what could have been but that is not anything new, for all go down the road of forgotten dreams, and endless failures, until one day largely by accident, we discover gold.

As I stood by the doorway, he said these chilling words to my heart, "If you are gay, I want nothing to do with you." Even though, after I was raped, even at an early age. I said in my heart, that I would never become something worst than what happened to me, and that was to begin to abuse children myself, because the world, and the church offered no solution for an out of a lost of control situation. That leads to a dead end. I made a covenant with God, that I would never sleep or as they put it these days, have sexual union with the opposite sex or with my own. I will wait until I was married, to a woman that could help me heal, and not a parasite, who just wants to feed of my wounds for her own ego, hence building her fantasy as you see with many modern day couples do, the husband the brave warrior, who goes to find food by getting a job and working 80 hours a week, to provides the luxuries of a fairy tale, that he neither has time for, and is too tired to enjoy it, thus neglecting his children, because he is the warrior of the modern day jungle, the Urban Tarzan as the wives meet in the park to chat dirt on their latest victims of woe and sorrows, and to build their fairy tale lives, like the play, acting out of, 'Cinderella,' who meets her, 'Prince Charming.' Instead, a woman that can help me heal the wounds of male rape as a child at the age of ten. I have now waited for 30 odd years. In addition, because the only thing my real father gave me, materially was a radio cassette. I had a choice between a watch and the radio cassette.

I chose wisely. I chose the radio cassette. I chose music to dance away the shadows of the monsters, which came from the phantom zone. At night to haunt me as I lay in my bed, with the cover over my head, to ward away the spiritual vampires, who came to drain me of any courage, that I had left, leaving me a cowering nervous reject of the modern urban jungle life, in the same place where the phantom of the Opera, the romantic disfigured musical genius, that dwelt in the passageways of the dreams of stardom, never really being recognized for his musical genius, like the X Factor rejects, and the many that the judges of fantasies directs into the Phantom Zone, the Paris Opera House, where genius go, disfigured by the simple facts that fantasies cannot be discerned from the real truth, they go into the passageways of Pairs, into the house called Opera, where the unreal sensation of being something, which can be touched, tasted, seen, smelt, heard but which is not physically present, the illusion of perception of light, which is hidden in thought as the French writer Gaston Leroux, in his masterpiece of literary writing of her alto ego resides, thus coming to life, and breathing into the wind of change, thus taking my imagination captive just as he did the young woman in white, in his fantasy. As I imagine that it was Saturn himself who was my phantom, and he wanted my virtue, to corrupt me, into a Beowulf, a warrior of lust, who slept with the Mystery Babylon as she cries out in her drunken sexual revelry celebrations festivities, "Come let us drink to the death of innocent, and virtue as I am corrupted, by my desires of touch, taste, smell, sight, and sound." From the very beginning as I go on the Crusades of the perception of light, reflected in the mirror of life, with the other (1096-1100 A.D.), Crusaders to gather myself a reputation, for barbaric stimulation amongst the Melodrama of a disfigured life, an inhabitant of the prison of life, gaining a reputation of appearing to be real but not actually existing, because in about 80 years or more, maybe even less, I shall be no more disappeared from the stage of life as I exit through the stage door of the theatre of existence, to be no more but a fading memory, I am like the grass as a flower of the field so I flourish in my youth, doing what I want, being who I want to be, and then as the wind passes over me I am gone, and the theatre of existence shall know me no more but only in the fantasies of the dreams of idol men as they remember the past, to hope for the future, never seizing the moment, instead not finding the horrific events of growing old, weak and diseased as decay eats way at their flesh in the form of old age like that which occurred at Ma'arra al-Numan. Proceeding the fall of Antioch, where the Holy Crusaders as they raided the countryside in the trimmed down winter months of one moment in time known as yesterday, thus in the absence of bringing anything like satisfactory riches for to be satisfied, what becomes precious, is what is of short supply, and as in modern times, it is the need for oil, they call it black gold, in that corridor of time, they needed to have food to feed their large numbers. It is the same as the British drinking themselves to death. The king sleeping with the Jezebel witch and giving birth to the he monster, Saturn, trying to give birth to his creature, the work of the flesh in men, all they do is have sex, and fight each other, the state of the living, both in the west, and some parts of the third world.

But you see the scene where she tries to sleep with Beowulf to bring forth her demon seed, is what Saturn does to the virtuous poor, and rich alike as he corrupts them with his demon seed, and this is the point, Jezebel can take on what they desire, because she understand the law of reflection, you can be everything beautiful to the eye but to the spiritual the light, they, the darkness, she always flatters you, trying to win you with her lust of life, to sell out your birth right her main, (Proverbs 5,) weapon is sex, and she seduces you, to love her for she wants the affection that only the Father can have from his treasures so long as the Father heart's desire, she thinks she has won, because it is a spear, that she is pushing into the heart of God, no man can defeat her, for she is a seductress, and will never give up. Is that why God is using mostly women and children in this last move of God? Those who thirst for worldly riches will fall, when Beowulf slept with Jezebel, the king gave him his kingdom, then he dies his curse of eternal dread is over but now Beowulf's curse starts, because he took the bait. Then he learns his mistake as many regret, when they become one with the beast, and her children or do something that they later regret, for the rest of their lives, Saturn never got that far with me. That is why by my intuition I told and wrote everything about my past with pornography.

If I Am Then I Must Be

Chapter 33

He that is Jesus said Father forgives them for they know not what they do. Therefore, he laid down his life, for even the vilest of creature, and even for the gay community who those who say they follow his teachings hate. However, since my father created the mess of my existence, and my existence created me, he had no right to expect me to give him grandchildren, when he had two in Jamaica.

I was no one's whore, if I am to marry, it will be of my own choosing, until then I will continue with my life, until I am delivered from it, whether the church likes it or not. For I know that the church is an institution, and at that point it is a nursing school, a nursery school where five year olds go. It is like a school where you learn the same things that people does. But at a certain point of your religious journey, if you can call it a religious journey, you leave school, and go onto university, and then you leave university, and then go onto your profession, if you saw someone who spent 50 years in a nursery you would think that something is wrong with that individual, and so it is with the church, and so not many have matured enough to leave the institution of the nursery church for the mature church, and that is the four walls of ignorance and traditional thinking and legalism, and go into the world, and be apart of the world, and learn to live-in the world but however, with the mind and heart and image of Christ and that is, "Father forgive us for hating the gay community, for being prejudice against another group of people that has as much right to seek for the truth that they may become like you, in their own way, and in their own time." But my father was not like that he was a prude, thinking of himself, and not us, and out of his love, and care from when he died, I only received about 1000 pounds from the sale of his home, which was nothing but yet, he wanted me to give him grandchildren.

However, I have forgiven him for what he did. In addition, that was to create me out of his one night of lust, with my mother, and then he was not man enough to fight for her against my step father, instead he went, and married a different Jezebel woman who only wanted his money, to fiancé her looser son and wife, from a different relationship. And when at the age of 28 I came to see him in his old age, just because he met my mother in the streets of Brixton, it seemed that he was more interested in my success, than his long lost son who went of to America, because his own father did not love him enough to even help him with his education, and up bringing, after all I had been paying my way through art school, and I was saving my money to better my life, a life that he created, and was never responsible enough to do his part as a real father, and support me as I grew up.

I on the other hand instead of becoming a deadbeat dad, like him I did not get involved with the opposite sex but instead put my head down, and worked hard, to better myself. But like a plague he came back into my life, and destroyed all that I had accomplished by making false promises, that he would support me, during that summer, if I came to see him, which I did, and as I should have known he betrayed me. He did not have a penny to support me, when I came to London, and he certainly did not have any money to help me get back to Boston, to continue my life far from his lies and fantasies.

Therefore, I lost all that I had worked so hard to build, while his second wife took out life insurance policies on her life to give to her children when she died, whereas he did nothing for me or for my brother, his first son Leonard in Jamaica, who was shot dead around 1995. I remembered getting off the plane, that landed in Boston just looking at what was ahead of me, thinking that I had worked so hard to put that kind of life behind me, and my own father again had betrayed me with his lies as he did with my mother, by getting her pregnant twice, and then abandoning her twice. I felt so stupid I thought to myself how I have fallen for the same trick that my mother fell for that created me, and my brother. My father's demon had brought forth a fiery dragon breath that he regretted for the rest of his life. In addition, in a paradox, it is the same with our lives as we grow old, we regret ever being born, and so we waste away in fantasies and delusions that come out of our hearts, that we are superheroes, trying to save the world, when the world is fine. It is just all those who think they are heroes, trying to save the world by blowing it up. As we see with many of our leaders as they change the way you become a member of the Houses of Lord forever. To allow the common person to be states men in this insane institution of privilege of exuberant riches, and titles that has no meaning to the common person. My father in the streets of Brixton, the streets of gold that is London, it was when I was in school, in America that he told my mother that he wanted to see me. In addition, when I did come, and see him, I watched him grieve as he realized, that she married him for his money, and not because she loved him, like my mother, and I said in my heart, that I was determined never to marry for money but for love, not for lust but for sincerity. I watched him go through every emotion possible, hate, anger, helplessness, sadness. I saw his tears as he cried cursing her, regretting not fighting of my mum against a devil's lust, for a naive woman who he destroyed for his sexual appetite, until my mother had to have her tubes tied so that she would not have any more children. The irony was that both my mother and father were played as they would say in American slang. 'They never found what they were looking' for as later I would dance, the dance of spiritual death to the U2 song, "But I still have not found what I am looking for." From the, 'Joshua Tree album.'

In a sense it was both my father's May-June my mother's jewel of Jasper as his first name found in the, 'New Heavenly Jerusalem,' coming down from heaven and the chamber pot my step father's last name that finally drove my mother insane, for she went mad with a broken heart, always ruminating that she spent her time trying to survive and not living. However, one thing she is proud of and those words of arrogance could not prize it from her, and that is she never abandoned any of her four children, that she had in London. One in Wolverhampton who had since died by drinking himself to death, and there in London oh how I used to hear her heart wrenching stories of families woe and struggles to survive in a world hostile to the poor. A world of unending differences to those who are less fortunate than others you would think that society would get the message not to mess with the weak. Not to kill the innocent, not to make money of their backs those who cannot speak for themselves and call it progress, because their shed blood will speak against you on the Day of Judgment. Oh how she cried when her only friend the only sister she could confide in died in her arms. At that point, she was alone doing her best to raise four male children. Chester had already turned against her. As I watched her cry out to God to ask why he was treating her like a whore, his own mother. He turned out to be the black sheep of the family. I remembered as we played as young children in our back yard at Talma road, how he would reaffirm with our next-door neighbour Ken that he did not believe in God. That we were not created beings, by a divine intelligence, and so he turned his back on creationism, even being one year older than me.

He was ten and I was nine. And as his father left, it seems like from an intuitional level, he blamed me for it all, and began to bully me with a passionate embrace, for he was really a coward, for when Neville who since died for what he was planning to do, and that was to crack open my skull, for calling him gay, which I did not. Chester my beloved brother was hiding behind the curtains in the front room watching, terrified as later confessed, "You have to be careful with those kinds like Neville. He is a killer, and will kill us, if you are not careful." As I stood alone in the dark cold chilly night, to answer his questions somewhat like the 'Ghost Rider,' as his flaming arrogance looked into my soul through my eyes, because he had a metal bar pole behind his back as he looked into my soul. However, I was innocent before man and God. Therefore, he received the full blow he sent for me.

His head went through a car windscreen, killing him instantly. You could say that it was a one of. Then Steven a boy at my secondary school also threatened me with a metal bar pole to impress some girls. He had the pole right up against my throat as I took the fighting stance. As he saw that I was serious, he backs down. Later in school that day, he said he was only joking. However, did not have the guts to apologize, and say he was sorry. When I came back from America, I left for the land of promise in 1980 and I came back without the promise in 1991. I found out that Steven had hanged himself in a jail cell, from another friend from school Mark with his belt. He was hearing voices like me. However, the worst one was Alan Goodrich he was a psychopath in my school. A short well built black dark skinned psychopathic liar. Who fantasized about starting a murdering gang like his brother? He wanted me to be his partner in crime. In addition, not because I was like him, I was the opposite of who he was, and was trying to be. It was because he saw a naïve child in me that he could build his fantasy

208

about being a gangster in and I had the word sucker written all over my face. Like all the relationships, I had since I was ten after my rape, until I was 42 years old. He would come to my home and tell me sweet little lies about how powerful his brother was as a gang leader, and on one occasion, he told me that his brother was shot in a gang related incident, and that we are going to be enlisted to fight some powerful gang. Now looking back on the incident, I can laugh with embarrassment.

The question remains how foolish could I have been to believe that any of what he was saying was true. However, with him and many others like him I wasted my youth being their slaves and being controlled by their egos. In a sense, I had broken free from my mother's image to be her old age pension. Someone who she would try and keep a prisoner to take care of her in her old age, which I do not mind doing but I am my own person, I will only help empower her, and not be her slave. However, to begin to experience it, with every relationship I had experienced for 32 years. Now I had broken free from the mental slavery of servitude to a dead way of life, that I am everybody's servant, and not my own. I want to be rich, powerful and well known. It had always been my goal since childhood, and these parasites kept sucking that greatness out of me. In addition, I would spend days, months, years ruminating on why, why. Now I have stopped all that, and I have found solitude where I can find time to investigate my life of woe and doom as the process of the resurrected phoenix begins to rise with all my wounds, seen from a distance, and a sun golden light shines from them.

It is the glory of resurrected image of Christ in me. As it draws those who the Father of all spirits has opened all their spiritual eyes to see them. Now I go on the hunt to find myself, and those who reflect me, to bring them together, to hear my tale of woe and doom. However, in that tale of woe and doom, the hope that came from believing in the resurrected image of Christ, on the inside of me, and them, and to divine knowledge and understanding. As they all drink from my well deep in the heart of the earth where the building blocks of all life came from as scientist are beginning to confer with the events of creation as written in Genesis chapter 1 and chapter 2, accept for the humanist. They are still trying to prove facts. In addition, my definition of an institution is culture and culture is from the past, and living the past in the present. Like the Jamaicans celebrating their cultural diets of high starchy foods and exotic fruits that were once used during the plantation seasons of old colonial Britain to help them stay healthy with all the hard work they had to do in the burning sun, now that there is no more plantation work as in working that hard to stay healthy. Most Jamaicans get diabetes, cancer, and so much more unhealthy diseases, and they in most cases put on so much weight, from celebrating a traditional diet. The poor working class poor in their ceremonial worship of their culture would eat fish and chips, fried in oil that leads to high heart disease. Therefore nothing new is discovered because all are contributing to what made the world chaotic, instead of trying to reach the ethos that Christ died for on the cross, and that is when the only person that loved him and publicly said to all, that he loved him. He abandons him in his hour of need and as a son his name is Jesus only came into this world to be loved by this world. In addition, the world could not even tell him, "We love you," by loving our enemies. Especially the church that say they represent the doctrine of Christ. Did Christ say on the cross, "Father forgive all those who do not practice witchcraft, homosexuality, the occults, and those who do, dam them to hell fire and brimstone." If the Father gave up his son for those who were considered unworthy, by God's standards should not the church give up it staunch on the gay issues that they are sub - human?

If I Am Then I Must Be

Chapter 34

It was a loupe warm day with clouds in the sky. Susan was feeling ill, it seemed like she began to panic as the childhood impressions began to resurface in a different form, trying to find a way of escape into her conscious world. It was like the childhood trauma had been masked, but not dealt with. However, temporarily forgotten because she went into shock, and her senses where suspended in time for half a century. She could not touch, feel or taste life, as most knew it. She only tasted like a jelly substance that the astronauts used when in space, suspended in time where there is no gravity, only a dark black space with pinholes, the stars shine through as millions upon millions of eyes pierced the darkness of her soul to look in. she was sick but not from any other disease of the mind. It was the concepts that she as a child internalized as her imagery friend in her illness.

The slaps were now called her best friends as she went from one abusive relationship to another with her two children who she had out of wedlock. Jack and Jill, and she named them after her nursery rhyme. Jack and Jill, in her fantasy, went up the hill to fetch a pale of water Jack went tumbling down, and so did Jill way after. The children Jack and Jill learnt from some of the best illusionists how to beat each other. Both were twins who learnt how to abuse each other, and their mother from the men folk that abuse their mother. But with the video games of world dominance, and mysticism, and hidden agendas surfacing in their conciseness to learn how to be psychopaths as they grew into the worst kinds of abusers those who abuse for money their own bodies as prostitutes. Jack's favourite game was, 'Halo,' at first he imagine himself as a Spartan secret name for Satan, just take out the, 'P,' and the, 'R,' and you are left with the name Satan.

He was one of the imagine orphans who had lost his parents in the attack on the earth from the hideous enemy, and so he volunteers to learn to be a Spartan, Satan's warriors to crush his enemies, his conscience made in fear. At such an early age, he wanted to crush the demons that plague his mind, and caused him so much pain as he heard his mother's cries of anguish as the men in her life would beat her, and then leave her for dead. How he would grieve in anger, as he knew he was helpless to protect his mother. Therefore, he would hate his sister Jill as she tumbled down the hill after him. He would take out his bravery as a Spartan warrior on her, by beating her up to prove that he was a man, not like those who abuse his mother but by hating what his mother had become in so he hated himself, and so he learnt to abuse like the abusers of his life, until he was old enough, mentally and not physically to abuse in the image of the abuser. In a sense he learnt to abuse by hating the abusers of his mother, then feeling shame, and despising his mother, and then blaming her for all what she suffered. However, it was the broken heart's way of life.

To hurt the ones you love, to try to control them, to try to mend them because you are a God of sorts. So in the broken home you see only control, control of the mother, on the son, and daughter, and then the son trying to control the daughter, and the mother, and the daughter trying to control the mother, and the son. Overall, all are trying to manipulate each other to bring out the best in their own image. In each opposite, which leads to chaos, and a complete break down of the family structure, and the more Jack, and Jill, and their mother tried to fix the situation, the more alien it became. The more they move away from the happy image of innocence, the three, and became the hideous three. Jack has to appoint in his frustrated life of how his family was not like other families that he would run away many times, and just hang out with the worst of characters that were considered so by the rich. He would hang with the drug addicts, prostitutes, and the worst of the worst. However, in Jack's eyes he saw them as God's treasures, when others looked down on them. The drug addicts, the alcoholics accepted him as a person. Even though he was a prince in disguised living amongst the poor.

Jack was instilled that he should have a job, before he gets a girlfriend. His mother Susan would beat this concept into his fragile conscience at an early age. In addition, the beatings broke his heart. He could not figure out why, if someone said they loved you then why were they are hurting you. This brought much confusion to Jack's fragile mental state as a young boy, and at every beating that he would get from her. She would say when you are working then you can have a girlfriend because then you would be able to support her. In addition, whoever she is, she will not be my burden or I will not be hearing that you are having money problems, like me. In fact, it was the only way she knew how to in still discipline into her fragile son. In fact, Jack was the only one out of her two children that she was hard on. This made Jack very resentful at her, and so he decided in his heart to break free from her mind control. In his culture, they called it witchcraft. However, in modern day medicine it was called mind control or more to the point, it is called schizophrenia.

As his heart broke, he would rebel against her partner in crime his stepmother. Because Susan's sister did not marry because no man wanted her, and she was a virtuous black golden-skinned poor woman. Who a freak caught having sex with a donkey back in her homeland in Jamaica, wanted to marry. And corrupt her virtue but his stepmother was a strong woman a determine woman, and she resisted this sub - human's advances, and so he put a curse on her, and her seed that she, her name was Linnet because now she is dead forgotten forever, and on her off spring, and that was Jack. However, this sub human freak went further he penetrated Jack's bottom with two of his soldiers of the damned because by committing this act on a ten year old boy. They were sentencing themselves to the hell fires that burned with brimstone, and sulphur. Sulphur is a substance that humans could not get use to, in the great mighty abyss of, 'The Lake of Fire,' where the damned make their abode. In addition, this would be the eternal home of all Jack's enemies, those who did not repent, and turn from their evil deeds, and accept Christ's offer of salvation. Linnet became Jack's stepmother, and so the curse was passed onto him. However intuitionally Susan, Jack's mother knew what she was doing, trying to save her son because she knew the horrors of being violated, and living in shame.

As she remembered how she was going to have her baby on a toilet seat, back in Jamaica but it was her nephew, Jake that took her to the hospital to have the baby, and it was a healthy baby boy that later turned his back on her, and was subsequently murdered. As he was a Police Officer and so, he was killed in the line of duty. John was her first born but because Susan moved to England, for a better life, he felt that she abandoned him, and when she came with Jack and Jill in 1974, the summer to Jamaica to visit them. He cursed her, and so sealing his fate, to die a lonely death. In all three sons of Susan, when she was in Jamaica died. In total, in Jamaica she had four boys, and one girl. Who became a soft porn magazine star in Canada, after she was tricked into going to Canada by a smooth talking con artist. She had no money, and to make money she had to strip for the camera.

But Audrey blamed Susan, and Susan knew it, in fact she knew that all her children blamed her for their failing lifestyles, and so, on an intuitionally level, she cut them out of her heart because she understood the human heart, and how cruel it could be. Jack's first love was Loraine, a young Jezebel woman that wanted a good job but spent all her time, after school studying, and sleeping around. However, Jack only wanted a friend. This was the period after he was expelled from his secondary school, for trying to burn it down. Eventually his social worker got him into another secondary. Again, it was a boy's school, and no one showed him any love, which Jack craved for. In addition, the main reason why he burned down his secondary school or at least tried to burn it down was that he was looking for someone to love him, and to treat him as a child. In a sense to give him, back his childhood that his mother so cruelly stole from him. Because he could not expect love from his mother, for she was trying to break him, to make herself an old age pension. Someone who would be so guilt ridden that he would spend his entire life, looking after her in her old age.

Many Jamaican mothers, who are now old, have tried it, and it has worked, on many of them. However, Jack was British, and he had the psychological make up of a white person and not a black person because his father was not around, to teach him how to grow into a black man. Therefore, Jack spent his entire life, breaking free from her control. To live his life, and at the age of 42, he finally realized what she was doing but he did not hate her for what she did to his life. He did not even care. He just said that he did not waste all his time breaking free from this mental slavery to go back into it. He said in his heart that he would help empower his mother but not care for her. For in her conversation as she got older she said that she wanted a servant to wait on her. At this point Jack could see the humour in her foolish ideas of what life was meant to be. As Jack walked Loraine home from the library, where they all met in a group, this was in Norwood near Norwood - library, it was up a steep hill. At the top of the hill turned around, and said in an alluring voice that her father was not in. In a sense, it was a hidden signal to come inside her, in her bedroom. However, Jack was not searching for the lust of the flesh. He was searching for true love. He was looking for someone to love him for whom he was, and not just as a piece of meat. This he never found. Because it did not exist, as he found out the cold truth that people need each other, and that is not love. Love liberates, and sets you free, like his love for his high priest that had set him free from religion, and its traditions. Loraine was very attractive in her school uniform. Her uniform was green, the colour of envy.

In addition, many boys of that school age envied the thought up relationship that Jack had with Loraine. Loraine was not that well built as in the heavenly dimensions in her figure. However, she made up for the lack of bodily features, with her looks. At the same time, Alan Goodrich introduced Jack to another attractive girl name Jean. Jean was very dark skinned, and had wild natural hair. She also had a figure. Jean would call Jack her boyfriend then play mind games with him. Jack could not figure out her game at the time. It did not make any sense to Jack who did not even realize that they were an item. However, Jean was very immature with her behaviour she was the kind of child that would play games until she fell pregnant. In addition, Jack was not into that kind of behaviour so he left her well alone. It was when Jack went to America to rebuild his life that he lost contact with Loraine. And then five year later, when he came for a vacation, to see his father, he could not find her, and no one that he spoke to knew who she was.

As Jack grew up, and became a man, in America, and not in England. He became a, 'Prince Charming,' women were falling head over heels in love with him, trying to get his attention but somehow he was not interested. Jack was still looking for that true love that he could settle down with and raised a family with but as his sister told him, when he met her for the first time that he was not moving in the right circles. At the time, Jack could not understand what she was saying but later as he grew in maturity and wisdom, he understood exactly what his sister was saying, and he saw it first hand. While in Denver Colorado, study photography, he met a secretary of the name Loraine, like his first girlfriend, back in London. But this Loraine was white, kind of an American Italian looking woman, and because she had a relationship with a black young male like Jack, the previous year, and it went well. She felt that Jack was sent by the Gods to replace the one who had left for his dream photography career. Therefore, she tried everything to get his attention.

The games of the weak willed defenceless woman alone at nights, was her best trick. But Jack had seen all these tricks from when he was a young man growing up in England, and he was not falling for any of them. With Jennifer Jack felt no spiritual love it was just physical attraction on her part, he knew that she wore a wig to church, and that what he saw of her was not her natural beauty, and so he knew that she was not happy with the way she looked in her own eyes, and so if God forbids, he would ever have the misfortune of marry her, he knows that all she would do is nag about her looks, not being up to scratch. For her it was the lust of the rotten flesh because she was a carnal Christian, a meathead, and could only think in terms of her emotions, and feelings. Jennifer was lusting after him always trying to get him to come back to her home, to meet her mother. Jack was most put off by her as she got to the church for Sunday service, she would change her shoes as she entered into the sanctuary of God. This practice Jack found very strange, and could not identify with it, he had never seen this practice in the non Christian world, only when his work colleagues would take their training shoes to work just to slip into something comfortable for the gauntlet that they would run at the work place as the starting line for the grand prix race.

To Jennifer, Jack looked good but however, she repelled him because he was spiritual, and she is non-spiritual. Jack became spiritual by all the harshness of his life as he grew up in a broken, and dysfunctional family. The unique thing about Jack was that he had hope, and his hope was very strong in him, and he drew like Superman his strength from the sun but Jack would take it one step further he would draw his strength from God's creation as he sat in the park that is Clapham Park, and would just marvel at what he saw God doing in the daytime, and sometimes at night, when the stars gave light to the dark creatures of the night. But both of them were from poor families. As Jack spoke with his conscious thought, this is what he said about himself, and the women that he had the misfortune to meet. "I knew that I was a dog and she would not admit that she was no better. Lachelle she was dangerous, she saw the potential in her boyfriend but she was not sincere. She hated her mother, and tried to use me as with many others to build her confidence in the wrong path.

She married for security, and because she hated her mother, when her husband hated his father for not helping them whose mother married a jerk because he was a doctor, and had money. Also looking at Jane as she is as with most middle class women in the church, offended by pornography you become what you hate, she is not comfortable with her own sexual identity, whereas those in the world who do not find anything wrong with sex are not offended with their own sexual identity, hence they have more healthy sexual relationships with their partners, whereas with Christians who try to put this image of taking offence with sex are actually giving place to the devil in their sexual union with their partners because it is based on a hate, love and shame relationship. They love their virginity calling it virtuous when in fact a true virtuous woman under the, 'New Testament,' is a woman who can talk freely about her pass as a sinful woman. After all Christ did not appear to a virgin, when he first rose from the dead it was a former prostitute who had repented of her sinful ways, like I did of mine with pornography, and I am willing to tell the whole world through my writings what I have done so that all will see that Christ has no favourites. He loves you all whether you are in sin or not.

Those who use their so called holiness as a crutch to trip up others from finding the truth, and that is Christ is no respecter of persons. The way he loves his Father is the same way he loves us all, these lost souls will never see the true, 'Kingdom of Heaven,' for it exists in the heart, and not in the stinking rotten flesh of our decaying corruptible bodies as they decay in the graves of our blindness to a saviour's love who died on the cross for all humanity even the gay community, if they will come to him, on his terms that is to rend their hearts, and turn from their wicked ways of sin, and accept his ways of holiness. Michelle said that both of my cousins were beautiful, hence, her pain was that she thought she was ugly, she acted ugly as a whore to a point, where one young black man had to hide from her because of her over sexual activities, based on her heart being broken by her fantasy boyfriend. Until she was fed up of it so she was looking for something different, same with Sadie, when I called her she spoke like a very angry and bitter woman.

Now she spends all her time hiding her shame of being a whore instead of bringing it to the light of her friends to be set free from her darkness The book of James let us confess our faults one to another and pray that we will be healed so we are so why bother? Doctor Smith knew me on the inside because she was a reflection of me but on the outside she was not me she said that I had many skills, and did not need extra training, and she was right. She said that I was depressed she was right. This is my question why is Saturn still trying to bring me back to sexual immorality it has and will continue to fail. And he knows this because he knew how I felt I would torment me in the form of me hating my aunt who I loved who kissed me on the cheek but yet she loved me, and I loved her, and that what I detests, which is love with being loved, which is just two animals rolling in the hay, he forced me to accept as his God, his pride and ego, when my aunt kissed me on the check, and all knows of mines as I confessed it to Sunny accordingly.

Then there was Janet full of pride so she projected an image of confidence in her soul, by studying social work, learning to drive, and choosing a field that required extra training. So she looks like what I desired as a child, 'Elizabeth,' from the, 'Tomorrow People,' which is the step before the new, 'Tomorrow People,' in America the program called, 'Heroes,' but on the inside she was very shallow as she showed with her key ring the key to her heart it said, "I am dam good." As a God you had to bow down to her image that she was dam good, before you could open her door to get into her house. I am dam good, if you praise me. However, she was not on the inside. However, Saturn allowed her to get me my DLA, which is based on the curse, and not based on the blessings of Abraham or Proverbs 6:30-31, Job 42. She used me as a piece of meat for her pride, which one to choose, and while at her day job she got angry when I called her saying that this is her day job, where she is queen."

If I Am Then I Must Be

Chapter 35

As I remembered the golden light of the shadow of the resurrected phoenix as she flaps her wings on those warm Sunday afternoons, after church as we sat down at 10 Talma Road in our part dinning room, and part kitchen. The air was like a classical musical song as the light intertwined with the Sunday traditional dish of roast chicken and Jamaican styled with rice, and peas, and style of how my mother roasted the chicken, was not in any Jamaican tradition as such but it tasted like Jamaican cultural chicken, and what made it so cultural was, there was love and fellowship that we shared with each other, and for our neighbours, our attitudes were one of respect for each other, I and my brother calling the woman who lived to our right, auntie Doreen, and the woman who lived to our left as Mrs. Benjamin.

There was a clearness of conscience, it could have been that we were very young, and did not understand how dark the human heart was, and is or could be that in those times we had so much light from the wings of the phoenix as the mythical creature flaps it wings, and the light of truth came freely into our lives, like a red orange that glows in our hearts. But now it seems that, that the mythical bird does not flap its wings anymore, for all I see is man lying to man, woman lying to woman, and the dark blend of black, and blue, the dark colours of our psyche reflected on our, the television screens as we escape into the illusion of self, into the illusion of self, strengthen by our lack of understanding, that what we are seeing others is a reflection of what we either hate or love ourselves, and so the dream lives, and becomes real, for when we try to change others, we are actually tying to change ourselves, it is the primitive prehistoric, and immature antidote of the Homo sapiens male, the final version of the modern man, and the only thing that I feel is missing from this creation, from the dark side of the darkness of our heart in our sub - conscious mind, is the understanding of what we have created as a spiritual building of our concepts that gives us as human kind the ideals that we so easily die for. It is called understanding but in truth how can we understand the dark black opaque colour of out id as it grows into a deep dark black opaque colour, like a moving shadow as we watch the cat trying to catch the shadow of the light as it runs in the light of our light of our light of what we call light that cannot be understood, until it is known for what it really is as with Hitler, and how dark his shadow was until after 60 years, after looking at the darkness in the shadow a newspaper, finally saw the light, and that was, 'if he had worked out his problems with his father, he would not have tried to kill half of the European people, in his mad pursuit to eradicate what he hated in himself,' until he killed himself instead of facing the horror of what he had done, and became, in the process to prove that he was a man in his dead father's eyes, it is like Batman becoming a legend to avenge his dead parent's murders because again Bruce Wayne wanted to be a man to prevent something that he could not change so instead of facing the truth, that he is vulnerable, he decides to dress up in a costume to prove that he is a man, and so with is with most men who cannot be intimate, and so they spend their time making money, getting drunk or getting a lot of women pregnant, and the most horrid, they battle out their egos, in the gladiator ring of the chip shop or on the bus, when they are told to be quiet, by pulling out a knife, and knifing someone to death, just like Batman or Hitler causes pain, and injury, in the pursuit of justice, that is their kind of justice because they will not let go of the hurt, and pain that they suffered as children, and now in their adult life, they wish to re - create the environment, that caused their pain in the first place, and so relive their fantasies, at the expense of other innocent people's lives.

Therefore, this morning while at Oxford Street Trafalgar Square, I met Nigel, Paul, and Mark, and another homeless young person. First, I gave Nigel my offering, about over 2 pounds for his ministry. In return, he gave Mark about 1:20pence. I prayed for Mark twice, by putting my hand in his, to heal him of Hepatitis C. He felt the warmth in my hand. However, I did not feel any heat. However, the second time I felt the anointing flowing from my hand, and he felt it too. I also gave them ten pounds, to buy phone vouchers for their phones. I gave them five pounds each when Nigel come over I was at peace. I said nothing but what was necessary I assumed, based on what Saturn had programmed me as in the song by, 'Linkin Park and Jay Z called Numb.' But I was not I just waited to see if it was a devil, that I was speaking to or a human being. I even thought I did not give him my phone, to make a phone call, I gave him something better five pounds each so they could make as many phone calls as they wanted, and Mark too. However, *as* I looked into his eyes, I felt the terror of the Lord for the first time.

The Holy terror of his nature, and I felt his anger as he held back his thoughts from me. And as the surfs hid their faces, reflected in their nature with their wings for Isaiah, for I perceived that this is not the of season to think on these things but to be aware, and they began to open up in the heart, and thoughts of the mind of God reflected the manifestation of the beginning of the manifestations of the hidden desires of the great I am. This is what I think or is a daydream, for this is the day of salvation, and I am the word of reconciliation to all men, creatures on this earth. For there is no difference between Jews, gentiles, and the church in Christ, and as Christ has ordained, that even the ungodly will see the kindness of God as was spoken by the Holy Angels long ago proclaims good will to all men.

Has any ever heard this proclamation, that resounds through all the earth, and it is written, 'though heaven, and earth will past away but my word cannot, I am the said word, to be done unto forever, I do not change I am not a man that I should lie nor the son of man, that I should repent, have I not spoken, will I not bring it to pass. Again, can anyone here this word of reconciliation that is spoken from heaven. Come unto me all those who are heavy pressed, and burden down with the pressures of life, and I will give you rest from your hard bondage, for my yoke is light, and easy.' I felt warmth in my spirit, while reading from the Messenger of the cross, by Watchman Nee page 14 lines 11 to 22. Thought sane, and wisdom manuscript, like Uncle Tom's cabin is preparing the world for judgment day, in the process of revealing their hidden secrets of the heart of man, to themselves as written in Ecclesiastes. 'Every hidden thing will be brought into the light, whether evil or good.' Exposed, and reproof the shameful things, that I do in the darkness. If our environment is not teaching us anything about ourselves, such as our desires, hopes, wishes and our dark natures.

Then we are not existing, and coming to the light of who we are, in the church they try to cover it up by trying to brainwash themselves in the belief, that they are holy, and that they are not just like any other sinner. The only difference is that they have seen the kingdom from a far but they are to afraid to take the spiritual path to get to the kingdom so they stab at those who are not like them, and who they cannot understand as a reflection of their own selves, in their own ignorance.

Then we do not exist in a state of awakening to the truth of who we are, our intent, and what we really have become, and so we force our limited perceptions of ourselves on others, and it they fail to see our limited perceptions, and accept them as gospel truth we remove them in the name of democracy, and freedom justifying our hideous, and murderous action, in the name of changing mankind for the better, and bringing freedom to all people, of all races and creed, colours, and poor, and rich in the image of our own image of the fallen God Adam, which is humanist creation of man in God. I mean, are you really setting a nation free, by killing all those who talk differently, and so create so much bondage, oppression, and fear, and injustice, by creating so many mental scares, damages emotions, starvation, diseases, the ending of the innocent fragile lives in such a horrible, and inhuman ways, and God instead just sitting down, and debating your difference at a table of friendship. Now is the season to reflect on pass failures, and mistakes by putting all the information, and knowledge gathered over a period of 42 years to decide clearly, which are the right path, and the right options to take. It is not a season for action until we are one hundred percent sure of what happened in the past, why it happened, and what is the best course of prevention.

I have noticed with the increase of dark activity also has come an increase of me, seeing the light, and been able to focus on the light, and to say no, and to stay in the light so I now know why Saturn has tried to increase his frustrations of darkness, it is because I am seeing more light of the id within me. *And the thing about* the control end in the churches is that when you give them positions of authority, they abuse it because, in the most cases, they have never succeeded at anything, no because of the stubbornness of their own heart, and their unbelief, that Christ had a better way and so, for instance, like ushers, it becomes their personal crusade to prove, that they are not failures so they dismiss what God is telling them, in their conscience so that they can be proven right, and if anything goes wrong, it is the devil, and not their failure to learn to love themselves, and forgive themselves by sincerely loving others, and forgiving others. And if they cannot love others, and faith works by love, then they certainly cannot please God, and if they cannot please God by loving, then they fail the test, that God is a rewards those who diligently seek him by faith so they are never rewarded by God because God only sees faith, and faith works by love, and if they cannot love other as themselves. Then they have never seen God, and they have no faith what so ever. So what they think they are receiving from Christ is from the devil of their own human reasoning, the manifestations of circumstances is in fact their own wishful thinking, and belongs in the realms of Adam's soul power, which is directly linked to Revelation 13:13. In addition, when these kind of carnal Christians hear a word of prophecy from God, saying what they believe will happen, it does not really mean it is that God has granted, it is just an observation of the facts, if we notice how David spoke to God, he was direct. He asked God if he would help him, and God gave him a direct answer, and that was yes in some cases, he gave instruction of how to win the battle.

Chapter 36

When I looked at the black art student with the name of J.C, which was an abbreviation for his full name that is, 'John Colin,' kind of like a the male pride of the, 'Mandingo Warrior Tribes,' of several different kinds of Americans from West Africa in American native form, especially along the Niger River Valley, the male animal pride part in the abbreviation of his name, 'John Colin,' shortened to, 'J.C,' the shorten version of his name made him feel like somebody important, while on the road going nowhere, when in fact in truth he was a nobody, a failure in life who through his own pride had failed so many times, and now he was on his last leg of the road going nowhere, and he finally has seen the light but just a glimmer of that light, and so with a defeatist attitude as he would look into the mirror of his own reflection in his more successful counterparts at the same time as he would call the entire staff of white teachers at our beloved art school in Boston USA racist, beloved because it was a state funded school run by the Boston State Department so it only cost in 1982, one thousand dollars to attend for a whole year, that is two semesters, and in British economic terms, it would be about five hundred pounds for the whole year because he was doing poorly in college, he would see his failures in his alter ego, like Clark Kent as a nerd, while trying to hide his secret identity as, 'Superman.'

He created his alter ego out of jealousy, for those who were doing well, and because he was doing poorly he poured all his darkness into their light, and so he began to develop his shadow of his alter ego so that he could fly like an eagle, only descending to grab his dinner for his survival, and that was the white female species because he thought they were easier than black chicks, and with black women they were only interested in living the, 'Camelot dream,' the fairy tale wedding, and the fantasy of bringing their children, into the world so that they could have theirs, and live their fairy tale story in real terms but never really understanding what true love, and commitment was, and how to be faithfully akin to one man as in the man they married, hence as supposed to the idol of the fantasy dream, that they are undergoing, and so at the end of their lives when they see their fake children, their fake marriage, their fake husband, they breakdown in grief, and madness because it was all a lie as they scream at their husbands, "I hate you, I married you for a fantasy, I did not love you." While with the white chicks, they just want to have fun, and they are easier. A black woman as I saw while at college in the states will not even associate with you, unless you could bring something of worth to the table of the debate, of the sexual union of the two independent halves, of one half, usually it is two halves of a whole but with black American women, in general they want their cake, and to eat as I saw as the black version of, 'Henry V,' as I walked around dressed like commoner, listening to their secret conversations, such as, 'wealth and manhood from a good stock.' I remembered my art school teacher, and how she loved my dedication to my art work, and how she would encourage me at that tender age but however it was when we went to see a famous Afro-American artist, that I inadvertently blurted out, about my training back in England, and when we got back to school, she took me aside, like a black American woman scorned, and scolded me by saying, "How dare you embarrass me in front of such a well known black artist, by telling him of your art experience, in another country, and not even mention what I did for you as your most recent art tutor?" I looked on in shock, and said that I was sorry.

But she never left it there she went further in her vendetta as she locked me out of the classroom, saying that I have to go to the office for being late. It was then I learnt about true American love, and what it really was a sexual, and lustful experience in, 'what can I do for you slut dog,' and so they become whores, and prostitutes to each other for a piece of the pie. Like John Mark's three sisters from Haiti, so madly in love with living the, 'American Dream,' that one married a famous a musician, and then the other two as they heard, that me and John Mark were going to start a production company, began to call me on the phone, and introducing themselves, like a sexual service as hostesses, "hello my name is Jane and I am John Mark's sister, is John Mark there please?" At times, you get sick of the flakiness in some young aggressive people who only see you as a whoring slut bag, to just lie down, and perform a sexual act for them. Even in the church while here in London as I went to a church near my home in Brixton dressed in my suite, looking all so sharp, eager, thinking, that this is my church at last and the senior pastor telling me to come, and see him, during the week. So I called him, and he did not even remember my name, and I told him what he said, and he made an appointment to see that same week so I go to his office, and sat down with him, and began to cry telling him, that I was sodomized, by two black gay catholic priest, in the church, in a satanic ritual service, to make me their host for Saturn's demonic witchcraft, and continue to the link between, 'William Shakespeare,' and, 'Hitler,' and he just said, "God can do it," and prayed, and told me to leave. He was no different than the whores, that I met in America, that were more interested in me as a fine specimen of male testosterone A well bred British Bull Dog, a perfect breeder to breed their fantasies into the American dream, and as I saw my own father die of a broken heart as he learnt about the Jamaican black woman who he married, and she married him for his money, and not because she loved him as his heart broke as he argued with her.

A dying old woman who worked herself to death, and gave birth to a stroke, that left her paralysed on one side, that eventually killed her, and when she was dead, he died soon after. They were no different, and so I closed myself of at the, 'New Testament Church of God,' in Brixton for eighteen years as I watched them admire themselves, thinking that they were blessed, when many of them worked in remedial jobs, shouting out from the roof tops, that if you worship God, the blessings will come down, which I found amusing as I wrote to the pastor's wife, and told her about what I thought about this ideology, that one person in particular was saying from the pulpit, and to addressed him, I said, "Is God a whore that if you just come with lip service, and sing some off keyed songs, that he would give you his treasures?" And then I wrote to the person in question, me being God, himself speaking to this person or fool, "If that were true then look at what I think of your worship, you are a bus boy in a restaurant." I never once had that attitude, and I still do not today. I never made any judgment about those who inflicted me. The thrones tormented my mind.

If I Am Then I Must Be

Chapter 37

Asking God was why people become sick even though I had never seen a sick person before, in my life. The sad fact is that because my ancestors had taken me captive, meant that I could not develop my relationship with the Lord of my true life. I also remembered being careful about what I said. If it was, a fantasy I made sure that I would confess that is was a fantasy, and not the truth.

Apparently, I knew the difference between what I said, and that it would come to pass, based on the revelation that I had received of the Lord Jesus Christ, I knew about sickness, and confession. All of this I lost in my ancestor's first attack against me. After my born again experience, my ancestors began to move in my life. After the first time I spoke to God, every time after that first experience I would mention his name something bad would happen to me, my ancestors had begun their battle against my life, to convert me to be like them, which still continues. Soon after a homosexual pastor from his mother's church, and his second in command met me, and told my mother, that I was mad because I kept looking around, a lot and that I would need to come to his home to be healed. He told my mother, that she would have to pay fifty pounds, which she had to borrow.

The night when I got to his home, he told him to get undress, which I did, and then he rubbed me down with some sweet smelling oil. After that, he told me to get into his bed naked, which I did. Then he also got into the bed naked, and he raped me. I remembered trying to keep his penis out of his bottom. He made sure he put grease up my bottom to make it easier for him to do his evil deed. I gave him such hard time that he said, "Why are you giving me a hard time?" After the experience, I did not sleep at all that night I remembered just lying there, looking through his window at the streetlight as it gazed in on this horrid act of sodomy.

Also at the age of ten while in my school's assembly hall, the children were having their daily prayer, and worship service. I asked the Lord Jesus Christ into my heart; this is what saved me through all I went through to break the witchcraft of my ancestors that two men who wanted power from them decided to agree to do to me, a ten-year-old boy. I did not see him nor knew who he was, that was how tranquil it was. I knew that I had received Christ even though I did not see him or experienced any manifestation in the spirit realm. It was by true faith that I had received a revelation of Christ, and he became a son of God. In addition, in the religious community a revelation is an idea or a thought that comes, that has no trace to the five physical senses. In addition, true faith is simply true and sincere love of God, not a concept of God that kills, and destroys individuals of their self worth, for a man in a cloth's idea of what God is like. And like a flash, I begin to write in my alter ego, like the mild mannered Clark Kent but this time I am Peter, the Rock of Christ, and my experience as I denied Christ when he most needed a friend, at his trial, and death, and resurrection. For me it was what I could not look at in the light of my own perception so I reflect on the truth in another person's eyes as so many of us, with mental illness do.

It was the same experienced, that Moses had when he saw the glory of God. This glory had kept him through his great imprisonment, by these spiritual ancestors. At the time he was attending Sunday school were Peter learnt about Christ but more so the devil. However, Peter did not recall ever hearing the name of Jesus mentioned in any of the services. Therefore, he believes that his ancestors purposely blocked his name from his memory, thus trying in to prevent him from receiving Christ as his Lord, and King. However, it did not work because he did receive him. Peter remembered at his Sunday school, his teacher kept teaching him in the class about the disciples of Satan who would count the odd numbers, and the children of God who would count the even numbers. He was trying to make a point about those who do evil are against God. This made a lasting impression on Peter, that even many years later he would not use the odd numbers.

Chapter 38

Peter was not moved by what his ancestors had done. That morning while he made breakfast as Peter consumed it he noticed a funny taste in his mouth. During the night his ancestors put many evil spirits on his flesh, one was the spirit of homosexuality, which did not stand a chance because the Holy Spirit was stronger, then anything that his ancestors could throw at him. Peter remembered every time, when this urge came on him, Peter while he was standing next to a male person, that he seemed to gain a strength in him, that overcame the impulses to act out this fantasy, that led to death, and eternal separation from the eternal creator. This evil desire came from his ancestors although he would not knock the gay community because being denied his social rights he understands, and even has understanding with the gay community on how his so called brethren try to deny the gay community their social rights as human beings for a written piece of paper that Christ did away with in his body of flesh on the cross of Calvary.

Another spirit was spirit that hindered him through all his adult life. It is called by the non-believer's schizophrenia. It was in the form of a giant spider's web. Making sure that he would fail at whatever he did in life. The second person that this ancestors used to abused him was his gay friend somehow he past on Peter's details to a man named Harry who was a painter and decorator. Harry was also a friend of the family who came all the time to take Peter painting with him. Peter had to stay overnight at this time where he would repeatedly abuse, and raped him The morning that Peter went home from this pastor's home as he walked up the stairs his aunt was standing at the top.

She had noticed that he was walking kind of funny, and mentioned, that he had sex with a man, which Peter denied because he was too ashamed of the event to even mention it to this family. However, they did not find out. Due to what had happened Peter turned his back on the church. Peter did not go to Sunday school again. Nor did he talk to God. However, he did not turn his back on Christ. Instead as his older brother began to play his tape recorder in the front room of his family home, he would go, and take the broomstick, and dance around it imagining, that he was fighting some unseen enemy Saturn. In this case, it was his ancestor Peter's ancestors were trying to gain access to his imagination, to try, and get him to worship them, which he would not do. Back in school, and college in America Peter chose art because he could not do well in any other subjects, that required him to use his mental powers. Instead, he had to use his imagination, which helped him to excel in the art to the point where he was given awards for these talents.

When he got to college Peter switch to photography, which he excelled to great level to skill. Peter was so good, that he could have became a famous artist but because of his teachers, and his past bullying by his ancestors, they stopped him through their jealously, they wanted him to come through them, and that they received all the worship instead of his true creator. By now he had forgotten about the church but not about God, Peter was still afraid of God but is it was the wrong God, it was the God of darkness, that he was afraid of that was Saturn, in addition, the sins that he was committing with pornography. His ancestors were successful in getting him into the crowd of the wicked. Born into madness he was an affront for destruction, a world of darkness. The poverty of his life was to fear living.

He could not die, he had not the strength to die but he live in world like a vampire's victim being fed off his fear. His desires were to live a normal life but the passion of madness had drawn him into a world of an argumentative story. It was like he was reliving his ancestor's lives. Life was devious it was like a sad story, to bring to his desire, to only have them explode in this, his face by the wicked people. Peter was in his own room fantasizing about being white. Having no father figure to guide him into manhood, he took on the identity of his television heroes, in most white people but sometimes Asian doing kung fu avenging their father's murder but this kind of fantasy save his life because he did not act like a black male but instead a white person because in the media black males were portrayed as criminals, and black woman as whores, that white men lusted after. Another factor in his deliverance from a life of destruction was the affects of the abuse but he would not realize this until later in his life. At the time, he was trying to break free from the traps of the abusers Saturn. Nevertheless, he could not break free because he was not strong enough. Instead, he closed himself of from the label, and lived in this fantasy world where he believed himself to be this white superhero, that was so vividly portrayed on television. In his mind he had created all kinds of heroes but every time he found himself fighting a very powerful enemy as he danced around his room, blinded by his madness, that he was white as he cried in pain, he called for his father in the bitter cold air as he walked home from work, and curse his step mother wishing her dead. He was blinded by the rage that was in him. In a sense, God had place a safety device within him that he could not strike out physically, and that tormented him.

Chapter 39

The cold winter nights warmed Peter's heart. They reminded him of how cold he had become. He would gaze out into the soothing night from his one window room, mediating on what could have been, He would think about the past with great intensity. He would go back to his childhood and remember when it was fun to be a child before his journey into the dark underworld of mental illness. He would remember the warm red sun as it belts down on him and his other three brothers as they played in his mother's backyard with the next-door neighbour's children.

He remembered a striking dark green tree at the end of the garden, that stood out in his strip back home, in his imagination. The tree was there as if to stop him from wondering too far from his home, in his heart. It is a long brown trunk, and branches, that grew from the main trunk of the tree. The branches had dark green leaves on them. This picture would always capture Peter's imagination, and he never knew why. Peter was shocked back to reality when the brother of the owner of the house where Peter lived came knocking on his door. Peter pampered, and wondered for a minute, that who would be knocking at the door of his fortress because he did not talk to any of the rest of the inmates, in the rooming house. He felt that no one was interested in a poor black boy from England who had lost his British accent, who lived in a room. Therefore, with great anticipation, he went to answer the knock at the door. As he opened Bob puts his head around the door and says to him, "I have not seen you around for sometime, I am just wondering how you are?" "I am fine," said Peter, Bob tried to engage him in small talk but Peter had learnt, that most men's intent of their hearts were to do evil, and he knew, that Bob was no different.

Then Bob said, "I want to show you the new changes that I have made in the kitchen," so Peter reluctantly came out of the hole that he had dig for himself, and went with Bob, to the kitchen. Peter was kicking himself because he did not know how to say no, when he knew what he should do, and that was say no. Peter walked behind him reluctantly. Then Bob said as he reached the kitchen, "You see I have put in new taps," Peter was not impressed, he would rather be in his fantasy world, where every thing is fine but in reality it would not be long before his world came crashing down. Peter said that it was fine. Then Bob revealed his true intent. Bob said, "I hope that you will keep this place clean in the future now that I have put in new taps in." Peter said, "I mostly eat out, and I hardly used the kitchen." Bob was shocked, and taken aback, a little because he thought that Peter was shy. Peter was also shocked at what came out of his mouth because, normally he would just agree with what he was being accused of, maybe something had snapped in him, and he did not know how to handle it. Bob said, "Oh I am sorry," "I am sorry, that you were wrong because I do not use it," said Peter. What Peter had done, was to build up a picture in his heart of being used, and abused by others, and that the pressure that came from his imagination had found a way to voice itself.

At this point Peter knew that something was not quite right with his mind, although he had not yet been diagnose with schizophrenia yet, in a sense it was a mask that he had worn for so long, since childhood. Then Peter said something else that shocked Bob even more. "I have to go because I am busy with my work. Goodbye." Bob said, "Bye too," and he walked back to his room, and opened the door, then shut the door, and Bob just stood there in amazement at what had just happened. He thought to himself how on earth did I get Peter so wrong. Peter went back to his room, and began to contemplate what he had done. He began to think that he knew, that there was some change in him but he did not know where it came from. Born into madness he was an affront for destruction, a world of darkness. The poverty of his life was of fear living. He could not die. He did not have the strength to die but he lived in a twilight world, like a vampire's victim being fed of his fears. His desires were to live a normal life but the passion of madness had drawn him into a world of an argument story. It was as if he was relieving his ancestor's lives.

Life was devious it was like a sad story to bring to his desire, to only have them explode in his face by wicked people, that surrounded him, like vultures feeding of his flesh of goodness. It tasted sweet in the vultures' mouths. People like John Mark that took advantage of his kind nature, and took most of his money to spoil himself on his evil lusts. The heaviness of darkness weighed him down, into a deep depression, which he knew nothing of. However, he would react to it violently, by smashing up his room or thinking on the things that evil people had done to him as he ruminated on them. His thought nature, until he discovered that it was depression. It was a black female doctor that showed him his problem with depression. He could not believe his nemesis was the instrument of his salvation because all through his life, his problems with the tall Dark female statute of figures, that came into his life, beginning with his mother. Now he had found a kind of freedom from that image that he had built in his inner conscience.

This kind of slender dark sensual woman now captured his attention. A multitude of love was flowing from her to him it was a love of a mother but also of a woman. Susan was the first woman, which he had let get close to him for a long time but due to his fearfulness, he would ignore her. Her eyes permitted him to approach her but he would not go to her. He was shy of women but in his heart, he wished that he were bolder. Peter kept telling himself that if he were not shy, she slowly not taking her eyes of him. She asked him how many were going to be in this function room tonight. Nervously he said he did not know. Susan was sensual and provocative as she was a dark satisfying slip into the luscious world of decadence. She spoke three different languages; French, Latin and English. She relish in the fact that her father was a persecuted Haitian that was imprisoned for his belief in Haiti. He was a lawyer who had strong political views about his government in Haiti. Her sweet delectable taste made men go mad as they approach the silk like body that stood inhibiting the viewer.

She would enthrone you through herself loving eyes and lips. Her appearance was very loud Peter never knew why he was attracted to her his ancestral spirits had trapped him into a world where he had no peace, a world in which he was meant to be alone waiting to be set free at their command. Nevertheless, Peter was meant to be humbled so that he would be grateful to his ancestors but somehow that did not work because civilization had matured, and now they have doctors, and nurses with medication, that can cure the mental slavery, that our ancestors put on us, which we now call mental illness. Peter was in a world where he was alone. It was strange how he could see the signs of his own destruction but could do nothing about it. He had no union with the opposite sex. His ancestors' image of him was of a gay, bitter man, heading for complete oblivion. To be completely forgotten by society until he would admit, that his African ancestors were godlike, in his life. However, since modernization had now come to the earth, Peter knew deep down, that he had no affiliation to superstition anymore. Not now, that he has a doctor, and a nurse to look after him. Peter had other plans for his life.

A good education, a wife, and kids, without a fight against the force, that thought, that they hold in his mind, that culture had put there through brainwashing him, into believing, into superstition, and old wives tales, that had no concrete evidence to support them The trumpet of war was sounded in his heart, it thumps against his chest Saturn's chest plate of dark evil, anything that was black was apart of that breast plate of Saturn's righteousness. He was delighted that he had realized what was causing his illness, the way he was brought into this world. The culture that had imprisoned him, his mother's ancestral roots. Peter would not tolerate no longer he was ready to free himself from the bondages, that kept him in his prison, dancing to fantasies, every night, in his one room but he fought, and resisted them with much destruction to his own self. Peter was a warrior, and music was his weapon of choice. Through music, he found a will to live as he discovered himself through the tunes that he would worship his ancestors with, each night in his dreams land, every time, that he would make a new discovery, a layer of the guilt would lift from his heart, and he would be freer to live the life that he wanted. However, his ancestral spirits knew that they could not confine him to fear, and they were scared. His ancestral spirits hated the modern world because many people refused to believe in them, and if they had no one to believe in them, they would become powerless.

All that would be left is the truth, which they hated. In addition, that was that humankind is in control of their destiny whether they would go to paradise with Christ or with them into the lake of fire. Peter met Susan while working as a waiter at M.I.T faculty club .Susan had just started to work there, while Peter had been there for a while, "My name is Peter what yours ?" "Oh it is Susan." Peter was brave to think outside the confinements of the thoughts that his ancestors had built around him, through his up bringing. In his heart, he knew that he wanted Susan as a friend. However, she was like a dark illusion that had no blemishes, a perfect sacrifice, a mass of matter that played with the wind, a flame that could not be put out in his mind. Susan asked him, "What do you do besides working here?" Peter replied, "I am a photography student at the Museum School of Fine Art. I am searching for my destiny through my art work." "That is interesting she said what do you mean by saying that you are searching for your destiny?" "Well each individual on the face of this planet is given to a mother, and a father for a reason. I have chosen to explore mines. In other words, I am looking for self in my artwork, the meaning of my existence. You see I have been labelled as a schizophrenic, for the rest of my life. It all started when I was raped by a minister, who practices witchcraft in my mother's old church.

That experience corrupted me." "I am sorry to hear that but how does being raped hold any bearings on your art work?" "I became an introvert, who could not communicate with words or academically. However, I was able to communicate with pictures such as painting, and drawings, then with photography. After the rape, I became a leper, in my own culture. The culture that God set up to protect me, and I asked myself, why I was born into culture to be segregated from them, to be an outcast. At that point, when I found out, that I was not going to be accepted, by them I came full circle. I realized that I had been living a lie. I came full circle with the battle, that I had to fight, and that is break free from the confinements of a dead tradition, that of my kinfolks used to honour their dead. I am not dead nor do I think that we should live for the dead. I want to find out why I am here. I want to, through my art discover, who I really am, and build on that idea.

I want to break free from the power that holds me captive, and find something to live for, and not die for my selfish and arrogant ancestors. You see after we are born, we begin to die, you see fear kills us. Some realized it but many never see what is coming, until they are dead, and they cry out for a saviour. Nevertheless, it is too late because they have entered into the black void, where all life goes, which have not found the truth. And I believe that the truth is Jesus Christ, the Son of God." His goodness that Peters had deep within his heart was diffused by the worldly lust. Nevertheless, Peter's true desire was to marry young to a beautiful black woman. A goddess of his heavenly Father's virtuous power of love, and compassion, that he would have been complete. However, his ancestors stole that from him.

A deep mysterious pattern evolved of seeking the false desires elsewhere in his imagination. The frustration of fighting his ancestors over this was great. Back and forth he would go, with these issues. One moment he would say in his soul, that this is what he desired, it is his life, and he will do what he wanted with it. Then like a bossy extension of his conscience, he would say the battle of his imagination, and his identity would begin. He would be consumed by these dark evil passions or would he come to the light, and live above it, that is his ancestors. Would he become a bitter gay black man, who could not communicate with the world, that his ancestors wanted or would he wait until he had freed himself from the chains of the mental slavery, that his ancestors had put on him. The choice was not hard from him to make. He would vindicate himself by saying that he was on a crusade, and he would exonerate himself, from what he was going through with his dignity. His ancestors did not care about his honour they just wanted him to worship them, in their depraved life style. He did not care about what they wanted.

He wanted honour in the eyes of the beholder, just as beauty is humankind's choice, based on their desires. What they will honour or is it a dark sensual feeling that controls them to make their decision about honour. It is true most of the moral world is against those who are gay but Peter was not because of his child abuse, he understood them. However, who are they to judge me, he thought to himself because their excrement is the same as mines, their blood is the same as mines. Overall, we are the same. All that is different is our mental appearance, and our outer shell. We think differently. We think based on our cultural heritage. Peter had broken away from his to form his own opinions, to make his own decisions, and choices on what he felt like. The backbreaking curse crushing him was more than he could bear. His efforts were vain. He thought he had gotten close to Susan but he was wrong. The true performance of their hearts was hidden within themselves, and like an electric shock, it came to the surface, although he met Susan, while working for the faculty club in Massachusetts. He felt he knew her before then. She was into the same things that he like, 'Astrology,' the, 'New Age Movement.' They like the same music. He thought that he could be her soul mate.

However, one thing that he did not have that she needed, like speech needs a voice, and that was money. He was not rich. He came from a poor family, and she knew it, she had the ability to sense people on a deeper level. She was a Scorpio, a mysterious and dark sign. It refers to when Jesus bruised the head of Satan on the cross of Calvary. All who falls under this sign were immoral, in a sense but very powerful people. Peter found out her feeling that she had hidden in her heart, when while waiting, for a function to end, for executives, he asked her, what she did, when she was not working. Nevertheless, he did this as a test because he new very well, that she went to Boston University, and that she was an undergraduate student there. She looks at him as if to say, how you dare ask me that question. Who are you to me, that I should tell you my own personal business? It was like something that someone had shot Peter in the heart, and he was in shock because it was a friend he trusted. Therefore, Peter went to the other side of the function room. To clear away the table but he could not clear away the distress in his heart, over this matter. Peter was sleeping when he had a strange dream. He saw a bed, and he was being pushed off the bed, the voices were those of his dead father, and someone's voice. The voices were telling him not to die.

He fought to awake from this paralyzing dream. He wondered why it happened, and what was happening to him. Maybe he was worshipping his ancestral spirits, and they were not pleased with his worship of them so they sent their soldiers to kill him. Peter could not figure out why this was happening to him, and it did not occur to him, to see a doctor. He was standing in front of a wall, in his apartment, when he saw, in a vision, a man proclaiming to be God. He gave Peter a flask to drink, which he did. After he had drank it, what was given to him, it made him very tired so he laid down to sleep for a while, later he felt a burning in his stomach. When he awoke, he heard three evil spirits in his room, talking to each other, saying that Jesus could not help him now.

Chapter 40

A white young man came up to Peter, while he was walking home from work, on a sunny summer day, and said high in his American accent, and Peter was puzzled so Peter said high back but reluctantly. Then this person began to talk about religion. However, Peter was not interested because he did not give his life to religion, he gave it to Jesus. What Peter wanted, was for Jesus to come, and take him away from all the pain, and hurt that he had suffered from humankind. New York was cold, and big. Peter did not enjoy himself in the big apple. Money was always a problem. The people were not friendly. In addition, this was because he did not grow up with them. In addition, he was British, the people he met were American, and they looked after each other.

He was isolated by his circumstances. He was an island in a great big ocean. At this point, of his life, he still trusted like a child, and that caused many problems. Peter was fired from a very good job because he trusted a fellow employee at the bank, where he was hired. He told her that he was moving back to Boston, after he had finished his training. He told her in confidence but she went, and told the manager. However, at this time of Peter's life, he could not be merciful; he did not see it from their point of view. The manager had hired a new member of staff, and expected that new member to be supportive to the bank. The manager called Peter into the office, and asked him, if this is true, that he was moving back to Boston, after he had finished his training, and could not lie because he was not brought up that way, said yes. Then the manager fired him. At that point, of Peter's life he was very resourceful.

He managed to get a job, working at fast food restaurant in Queens, which did not cover his rent, and he could not stay with his cousins, whom he originally moved to New York from Denver to be with because he had moved out of their apartment. He could not stay with his alter ego that had been damaged through the abuse that was done to him. All became an enemy to him, through his imagination. He wanted so desperately to be by himself so that he could grieve at the lost of the years, that he spent being abuse by a system, that was not real. He was a part of the environment, that he came from and he wanted to examine that environment to build a new man just as his mentor the Lord Jesus Christ came to earth as a man two thousand years ago to examine the depravity of his creation's soul so that he could create a new creation, him being the first raised from the dead, out of the dark void of the human experience in the earth, a new him. If he had no environment to be apart of he felt that he could see his problems more clearly. However, before he moved to his last home in the Bronx, he moved into a hotel, that was close to where his cousins lived. It was George who worked with him at a super store in New York City that introduced him to the owner of his apartment that he rented, and could not afford to pay the rent on. Because Peter had no sense of reality he could not for - see that he would get into problems with the rent. George told Peter of an one-bedroom apartment, that was available in the Bronx for 350 dollars a month. Peter was interested, and he put Peter in contact with the property owner, although it was more than he could afford.

It was an a typical winter morning that he met Mr. Fist. As Peter walked into his office, he was greeted by Mr. Fist with a handshake. His eyes pierce Peter's soul violently, even though he was civil to Peter. Peter could not sense any hostilities behind the front that Mr. Fist was giving him. He seemed to be very pleasant but that was the greed talking. It was the aura that he gave in the office. They both talk to each other for a brief moment in time. "Good morning," in a sharp voice with a confident posture, sitting in his chair, Mr. Fist said. Peter replied to his sign of a false friendship. Peter had wondered if he had become a victim of Hollywood, the pride of the wasp, Beelzebub. It is when we see too many good role models of the wasp in the media that they believe it is so, and so they become arrogant, and prideful, which leads to them making mistakes. Peter began to think abstractly as his nerves began to take over, pushing him into his alter ego. Although Peter knew, that it was Satan who had destroyed his life to make him his vessel of death as the reincarnation of, 'William Shakespeare,' who was born in 1564, and Peter was born in 1964, like Abraham Lincoln, and John F. Kennedy being shot in the back of the head one hundred years apart. Peter was born four hundred from the birth year of Shakespeare, and Peter understood the spiritual labyrinth, that he had been negotiating all his life, Satan trying to be his God, when he originally gave his heart to Jesus Christ. But Peter had discovered what Satan was up to, and had caught him in his act of his deception, and so now that the thief had been found he must restore sevenfold to Peter's life. He learnt from his experiences, in the occults about demons, and Satan who he called Saturn, and he was wise enough to know that Satan, and his demons even though they are real but to humans, they are a myth, which is a true reflection of what they are. He learnt that in order for something to be real and to be true, you must understand it. In addition, to understand something, that is that evil, you must be it. If you are not it, you cannot, from a human perspective, to know what you are doing, and he has seen many in the church who arrogantly boast, that they can tell us, and teach us about beings, that are so dark, and evil, when in fact all they have to go on, is just an experience, a reflection of an entity, that is so dark, and twisted.

While he was sitting on the sofa, outside his apartment, he heard a young man beating his carpet on the stairs then all of a sudden, he heard that person shout out, "No, no, no," as he ran back to his apartment. He did not know what Satan's demons were doing to this poor soul, and he was yelling, and running in terror. Peter said to himself, "I am a Christian who likes to think about God a lot, and to do his will on the earth, whatever that might be. The reason why I say this is because I do not know the whole bible so I do not know everything that pleases him. I am also a man who is learning to live with my disability, in the hope, that one day I will totally heal myself from it, with my faith confessions, which is beginning to happen, and everything that Jezebel stole from me, and my family for over two hundred years, to force me to build her church, will be restored sevenfold. I now understand what the apostle John saw of you and why the angel that stood with him as he gazed on you as you did your filthy practices from your womb giving birth to them through your birth canal, which is called, 'Pandora's Box,' that smells so bad, and why the angel asked him why he was looking at you so hard, at you in your orgies of sadomasochism as you rubbed your joy stick with sand paper for the extra feel as you are part man, beast, and woman as you masturbated in the dark, where you thought, that no one would see you, and what you do, and really are, you notorious, nasty, smelly slut dog. It was because of what he saw you doing in the dark in your den of iniquities of your orgies with your fellow demons as a slut bag that you are. I am kind, and generous to all those whom I meet in life. Firstly, I am an artist, and

I like to express myself with photography but due to fear creeping into my life, like a parasite, that has hindered me I am paralyzed by it because I like to live by faith. I am able to hold my own against fear that is trying to consume me. One of the ways I like to deal with my fears is to help the poor with all I have. I like to watch programs about faith, and people of faith so that I can learn from their mistakes. In addition, I like to pray in the heavenly language, that my Father in heaven gave me through his Spirit. Nevertheless, most important I like to talk to God about why his creation will not come to him, especially in Europe; and why they love death more than life, you have teenagers drinking themselves to death, and you have an HIV disaster about to hit the world, like rock from the heavens. You have violence, and crime growing to an all time high. People are living in fear of one another, killing each other for an idea, that they are God. And yet our heavenly Father still loves them, and us; that he would send his only begotten son to die on the cross in our place so that we might be able to come into his presence. Furthermore, I am a man with a powerful singing voice that I believe that God made. My desire is to sing the old Negro spirituals about Jesus. My goal is very simple I like to live in peace with God and man. I love all people even those who have, and will do me wrong. What I would like to happen is that God comes to the earth, and heals the nations. And teach us his ways, and show us his path, and not the church who say they are called by his name but all they do is bible bash us, the sinners." And he kept saying these words to Satan, and his demons telling them, that he would not build Jezebel's church in the earth. So she killed five of his family, murdering three, which are now in hell with his father.

Chapter 41

Peter was in his room fantasizing about being white. Having no father figure to guide him into manhood, he took on the identity of his television heroes, mostly white characters but sometimes he fantasize that he was an Asian poor boy studying kung fu to avenged his father's murder. Since his father was not around, when he was growing up, which was the underlying source of his illness, this particular theme was very popular with him.

Peter would not come to the realization, that he was the product of a one-night stand, and not out of true love, and these ideas his adversary forced on his fragile mind so that he would one day betray his Christ seated on the throne of his heart, and build the Jezebel slut bag's kingdom on earth, which would have led to the death of millions as he saw her work in the media arts. When television programs like, 'House,' that featured uncontrollable diseases, that are life threatening, he knew what the notorious slut bag was up to as she breeds her filth into the hearts of those who would watch this kind of filth, on television, and enjoy it, not knowing that the heart is the spiritual breeding ground for the work of Jezebel.

So he knew in the future that uncontrollable diseases were going to break out in the earth, like the Bird Flu plague, which is just the beginning. He saw also the revenge movie syndrome so he expected Jezebel to create in the heart of man the ethos for revenge, which leads to murder, rape, and other horrid ways to die. Satan tried to program Peter through, 'Hollywood,' by creating his life as he did with so many lives on the media screen, this was Jezebel's territory, where she excelled in her fantasy of being a queen, that is worshipped as a Goddess, when in fact she is just a smelly whore bag out of the region of hell, in Peter's eyes as he grew up in her world of the spiritual labyrinth of fantasy films of revenge, and of saving the world. He would have been the perfect hero, handsome, intelligent, honest, humble, and loving. This is what Jezebel, he thought the slut bag had her orgasmic moans, and groan in hell as she gave her king, that is Satan blow jobs, that caused even him to moan like a whore, in heat. The main attraction to Peter was the struggle, that the main character would face in learning their art to avenge their father's death. However, these kinds of fantasies save his life from harm because he did not act like a black male but instead a white person. He did not look for love in the bars, and so on; instead, he looked for love in his fantasies. Peter was happy to live in his imagination, which is the strongest part of him, at that time, and is still the strongest part of him today. However, that he is a committed Christian now, and he finds it difficult to change the images, that he built up in his imagination to godly ones, although he had the good behaviour of a white person, and the focus, which was really because of the abuse, that made him into a shy eunuch, that could not use his God given abilities to further his life. Instead he always failed at what he did because he was not sharp in his thinking, which led to him making the wrong decisions, also because of the sexual abuse, he was ashamed, and felt that he could not trust people but that changed as he grew older, and learnt to control his thoughts. He did not steal, nor was he a player with the women because in the media black males were portrayed as criminals, and black women as whores, that white men lusted after, especially in America.

In addition because these were the role models, given to the poor, they would imitate these images. Nevertheless, Peter was different, he had ambition, and he wanted to be someone important. In a sense, Peter had hope, which most other poor ghetto kids did not have. Therefore, Peter was willing to suffer in silence, and to be patient, and wait for his freedom to come, from the constraints of his ancestor's prison, and when he went to buy his first record to play on a mini record player, that his primary school teacher gave him, for being a well-behaved boy in class. Peter bought a record by Earth Wind and Fire. His next-door neighbour was shocked when he learnt of Peter had done, and took him out to a black record shop, and bought a black produced reggae song. This was the type of control, that Peter tried to get away from all his life but because he wanted to be accepted, he would always end up in this kind of group, which left him bitterer than the previous encounters, also because slavery had destroyed the will of the black people, and their heart. Poor black people were victims. Peter had learnt many years later, while living in England, that scientist in the US Army around 1993, had taken blood from a man, and placed it into a container. Then the scientist placed a lie detector devise into the blood, while the man who's blood was in the container was watching old war films. While the man watched the films, when he got agitated, the detector machine would go wild. In addition, what the scientist found out was that the blood in the container reacted the same way the man did while watching the films, although the blood was separated from the man who took part in this experiment. It all had something to do with the white blood cells. At this conjunction in his life, he knew that most of his problems were because he had been contaminated with the blood of his ancestors, vs. the blood of his saviour, Jesus Christ.

At last, he began to understand the struggle in him that created so much confusion. Nevertheless, what Peter realized, was that through that struggle, he learnt who he was, and clarity of mind came to him. Even though he was labeled with schizophrenia, his mind, through all the mental torture had grown and matured. In a sense, he was like the Phoenix born from the ashes, and fire of a very destructive beginning in life. The black male father figure would not be around to look after their families because, during the days of slavery, the white owners would use them to breed their black women, and when they had children, the black male would be moved on to another farm, and so on. Therefore, Peter was not alone in the realm of the absent father, in the black western culture. In fact, he was shy of women. In addition, to enlarged this theory in his life was what his mother said to him when he was very young and that was, 'not to have a girlfriend until he had a career and could afford to look after her.' These words had a deep impact on Peter's life because he always wanted a companion but because of the curse his mother put on him, he could not have one until the prophecy was fulfilled. At the age of ten, before he was abused, he was always thinking about the kind of woman he would marry. In fact, he would go to bed at night, and dream of her, and their children.

Lightning Source UK Ltd.
Milton Keynes UK
27 September 2010

160414UK00001B/28/P